MORE THAN MEDICINE

WITHDRAWN

MORE THAN MEDICINE

the broken promise of american health

Robert M. Kaplan

Harvard University Press

Cambridge, Massachusetts
London, England
2019

First printing

Library of Congress Cataloging-in-Publication Data
Names: Kaplan, Robert M. (Robert Malcolm), 1947– author.
Title: More than medicine : the broken promise of American health /
    Robert M. Kaplan.
Description: Cambridge, Massachusetts : Harvard University Press, 2019. |
    Includes bibliographical references and index.
Identifiers: LCCN 2018024768 | ISBN 9780674975903 (hardcover : alk. paper)
Subjects: LCSH: Medical policy—United States. | Preventive health services—
    United States. | Medicine, Preventive—United States. | Public health—
    United States.
Classification: LCC RA395.A3 K353 2019 | DDC 362.10973—dc23
LC record available at https://lccn.loc.gov/2018024768

For the family that questions: Margaret, Cameron, Seth, Ashley, Oscar, and Rose

contents

MORE THAN MEDICINE

Introduction

Apparently, nothing is more important to Americans than good health. That is why we are willing to spend so much to achieve it. Health care now accounts for the biggest sector in the biggest economy in the history of the world. In 2017, the United States spent $3.2 trillion, or about 18 percent of the gross domestic product (GDP), on health services. Most countries that Americans consider our economic competitors spend less than 11 percent of their GDP on health care. If the US health care system were an independent country, it would have the fifth-largest economy in the world, behind only China, Japan, Germany, and the United States itself.[1]

One reason the United States spends so much on health care is that it is deeply invested in the most expensive variety of that care: biomedicine. Advocates for this sort of care have a compelling argument on their side: more investment means more medicine, and more medicine, the argument goes, means more cures, greater longevity, and increased quality of life. The validity of this argument is obvious to Americans, and why shouldn't it be? We know that diseases result from malfunctioning biological systems—infections, organ system dysfunctions, toxic exposures, accidents, and genetic abnormalities. To identify aberrant biological systems, we need biological tests. To fix these systems, we need pharmaceutical interventions, medical devices, and other therapeutic techniques directed at the biological system. The faith on which American health care is built is that basic science can be translated into miracle cures, rescuing patients from the grip of life-threatening illness. Indeed, we hear stories of such patients frequently. They inspire us to not give up hope—and to spend without limit.

The narrative of miracle cures surfaces everywhere. It is in advertisements for pharmaceutical products and hospital services. Charities push it in solicitations for contributions. Doctors and patients talk about great new scientific accomplishments and those on the horizon. Researchers justify their budgets by promising curative medical technologies. For instance, in 2014, National Institutes of Health director Francis Collins told the Senate Appropriations Committee that NIH scientists had brought down the US death rate from coronary disease by 60 percent and stroke by more than 70 percent compared with the three previous generations. Credit went to their work on heart attack and stroke prevention, cholesterol-lowering drugs, blood-pressure-control therapies, and innovative strategies for dissolving blood clots. Collins closed his testimony with the story of Nic Volker, a 6-year-old from Monona, Wisconsin, who survived a mysterious, life-threatening intestinal disease with the help of NIH-funded biomedical research.[2]

It is no wonder, therefore, that biomedicine dominates federal research expenditures. In 2017 NIH spent about $33 billion on biomedical research. By comparison, the National Science Foundation spent just $7.7 billion to support basic research in all other areas of science combined. The cure narrative also shapes decisions about how biomedical-research budgets are spent. Grants identified with the search terms "genome," "stem cell," and "regenerative medicine"—all research areas associated with disease detection and therapy—consume 57 percent of the NIH budget. Between 1974 and 2014, the number of indexed biomedical research articles grew 410 percent; the same period saw a 2,127 percent increase in articles identified with genome research.[3] Meanwhile, faith in cures, and the large budgets thereby justified, attracts young minds to biology and medicine, starving other fields of talent and financial resources. That same faith fuels runaway prescription drug prices: only because we believe we need them are we willing to pay so much for them.

In this book, I ask an unusual question that would be much more common if we were not so invested in the status quo: Is it worth it? Medical science has undoubtedly made great advances. As a medical researcher and science administrator working in academia and government, I have been fortunate to witness and take part in these advances. I have seen the injured healed and the sick made well. But are we getting the return our investment demands? In the chapters that follow, I argue that we are not.

A Critical Look at Biomedicine

We need to rethink our basic approach to biomedical research and health care. As practiced today, our approaches are too expensive and too often fail to make good on the promise of providing cures. They also rely on a fundamentally mistaken, mechanistic view of the human that diverts attention from the kinds of research and intervention that would be most useful in improving Americans' health.

At this point it would be folly to deny that American health care is enormously expensive. What we don't often recognize, though, is that spending the most doesn't necessarily make for the best outcomes. Americans have shorter life expectancies and higher infant mortality rates than the people of most other developed nations, and the gaps are widening. The disparity is present even among the most privileged: the death rate for US white non-Hispanics between the ages of 45 and 54 is nearly twice the average for whites in that age group in Sweden or Australia.[4] On the whole, the United States ranks last among rich nations on key indicators including life expectancy and probability of surviving to age 50.[5]

Of course, some Americans can afford excellent, cutting-edge health care, but even this is often less impressive than it seems. Recall NIH director Collins's claim that biomedical research investments are responsible for dramatic declines in death from heart disease over the course of generations. Although new medications have helped, a review of more than fifty studies indicates that at least 50 percent of the mortality reduction is attributable to nonmedical factors.[6] For instance, a major source of the drop in heart disease deaths is declining tobacco use.[7] The course of the heart disease epidemic closely follows that of cigarette smoking's popularity. Smoking was relatively rare in turn-of-the-century America; its incidence began increasing around 1910, plateaued in 1945, held steady, and declined in the 1970s. Similarly, incidence of heart disease began rising in 1910, plateaued in 1945, and fell after 1970.[8] The rapid decline in deaths from heart attacks and strokes began well before patients had access to modern heart medicines such as cholesterol-control drugs.

Indeed, there is little evidence that advances in drug therapies have saved people from heart disease. In the past twenty years, the most credible major randomized clinical trials to evaluate treatments intended to reduce premature deaths from heart disease were sponsored by the National Heart, Lung, and Blood Institute. Their studies have high credibility because they monitor conflicts of interest and they require the highest standards of transparent reporting. Of the twenty-five treatments tested in these high-quality studies, just one was associated with significantly increased life expectancy.[9]

And yet, testifying to the power of the cure narrative, Americans believe we have the world's best health care. A 2013 YouGov public opinion poll for the *Economist* asked Britons and Americans, "How do you think the US compares with other wealthy countries, such as Britain, Canada, France, and Germany?"[10] Respondents were asked to compare the United States and these other countries in terms of life expectancy, infant mortality, obesity, and homicide rates. As I explore in Chapter 1, the United States has lower life expectancy, greater infant mortality, and significantly higher prevalence of obesity than these other countries. The number of homicides in the United States is also far greater. But US respondents told poll-takers the opposite for each category. In response to each question, US respondents reported that their country had superior outcomes. In other words, Americans downplay poor outcomes and fail to account for public-health concerns that can't be solved by cures.

Our tendency to impute great power to a system driven by medical interventions, and to deemphasize the effects of social and behavioral risk factors such as obesity and homicide, reflects widespread misunderstanding of the people being cared for. Medical science in America today treats people like auto garages treat cars. Is your oil low? Add some. Is your hemoglobin low? Add some by taking medicines that raise it. Just as mechanics remove and replace malfunctioning parts, surgeons remove malfunctioning organs and sometimes replace them with transplants. This "find it and fix it" philosophy works for some health problems, but not for all. Treatments may improve some physiological measure while having no effect on longevity or overall health. They may be harmful as well, producing serious side effects.

Meanwhile, over-focusing on biological mechanisms directs attention away from the many social and behavioral determinants of good and ill health. Current biomedicine recognizes the quality-of-life and longevity effects of violence, poverty, racism, workplace policy and stress, and poor education. But the current practice of medicine pays very little attention to these influences: they cannot be easily addressed with medicines or surgeries.

Taking Control from the "Dead Men Ruling"

Effecting change in public policy is daunting. Citizens often clash over spending priorities, whether they want more funding for schools, infrastructure, law enforcement, health care, or any other public project. Many citizens also want spending cuts and lower taxes. And lobbyists push for their industry's bottom line, heedless of governance philosophies or the greater good.

Yet it is not just good-faith disagreement and bad-faith profiteering that are to blame for unwise spending—too much for things we don't need, too little for things we do. As the economist Eugene Steuerle shows, many of our investments are just continuations of previous ones.[11] Programs, once established, develop lives of their own and can be hard to dislodge. Spending priorities set in one year often persist to the next, and the next, and so on down the line. Although these programs live on, they often represent the priorities of people who are no longer alive. In other words, Steuerle explains, dead men rule.

The ideas governing current scientific research spending are mostly those of dead men such as Vannevar Bush, the engineer and public administrator who pressed for the creation of the National Science Foundation. Once programs are funded, advocacy groups form to keep them in place. Scientists in nearly every discipline lobby hard to assure funding for their research area will grow, or at least stay the same.

The rule of dead men has not encouraged us to be stingy, but it has directed expenditure narrowly toward biomedical research and intervention. Compared with countries that enjoy better health outcomes, the United States spends significantly more on medicine and significantly less on other human services.[12] This is not to suggest that spending on biomedical research and health care is always wasted, but there is reason to believe that a different allocation of resources, toward social services and away from medicine, would produce better health outcomes.

The Science of Better Health

In many parts of the world, scientists and citizens concerned about rational, well-developed policies must contend with challenges from pseudoscientific and anti-science forces. The United States is no exception. Highly organized and richly funded pressure groups contest well-established evidence of evolution, the causes and effects of human-generated climate change, the benefits of vaccination, and the contributions of social science. It is obvious that risky sexual behavior increases the chances of serious infectious problems including HIV and hepatitis. Yet, serious efforts have been organized to block funding for research on sexual behavior. And, during an epidemic of deaths associated with guns, restrictions have been placed on the Centers for Disease Control for studying firearm-associated deaths.[13] One might worry that challenging the cure narrative, and the value it assigns to biomedical research and medical care, is just more science bashing.

But what I have in mind is not science bashing at all, but science practice. I use evidence reported in mainstream peer-reviewed biomedical literature to inform hypotheses and policy ideas. My arguments are not outlandish. In fact, most physicians and public-health scientists are familiar with the position I take throughout this book; they discuss related matters in journals and at professional meetings.

I hope you will see no disconnect between my arguments and the science you can find regularly reported in the leading medical and public-health journals. Instead, the disconnect is between professional and lay understanding. My goal, in part, is to help the public appreciate what many scientists appreciate already: that the dominance of biology and medicine in American approaches to health care is a source of dysfunction. Faith in cures costs us massively in terms of direct expenditure and in terms of opportunity. By sucking up resources and diverting attention from social and behavioral factors, the cure-driven biomedical system hollows out our ability to provide human services, leading to worse health.

In fact, it is our current course of action that lacks empirical rigor and method. To continue would be to engage not in science but in insanity, according to the definition famously attributed to Albert Einstein: "doing the same thing over and over again and expecting to get different results." In the chapters that follow, I explore why this is so, showing why public faith in cures is misplaced and indeed dangerous—and how nonmedical investments can do more to improve the health of all Americans.

1

Let's Be Average

The year 1945 marked the beginning of America's "war on disease," an idea dear to Vannevar Bush, who originally proposed the development of the National Science Foundation and who led American science efforts in the 1940s. Bush proposed to further the remarkable progress in life expectancy witnessed between 1900 and 1940.[1] That period saw large declines in the incidence of yellow fever, dysentery, typhus, and other diseases. Bush attributed these achievements to the biological engineering ongoing at the time, which gave us vaccines, penicillin, and the insecticide DDT. Even more remarkable was the 0.5 percent annual increase in life expectancy reported each year between 1940 and 1945.[2]

Many of the treatments that lowered mortality rates in the first half of the twentieth century are now regarded as primitive, even harmful. And there wasn't much access to care during that heady first half of the 1940s, because about half of physicians were involved in the war effort. Yet the increase in life expectancy during the first fifty years of the century was greater than that of the second fifty. Between 1900 and 1930, when essentially no modern medicine was available, US life expectancy increased by about 3.1 years per decade. Over the past thirty years, it has continued to increase, but at a much slower rate of about 1.5 years per decade.[3] And for some demographic groups, life expectancy is now declining rather than lengthening.[4]

One might point out that initial gains tend to be easiest: early on, there is a long way to go, and, once the basic problems are taken care of, every marginal improvement is harder to achieve.

But this does not exonerate Americans' faith in—and spending on—biomedicine, because the biomedicine we have today was not responsible for the early gains that so impressed Bush and his contemporaries. And if there is some limit to human longevity that can be approached only asymptotically, at ever-escalating cost, then we must at some point question whether that cost is worth paying.

Even so, the war-on-disease narrative that began with Bush and his ilk remains attractive, and it appears that Americans are ready to continue the fight no matter the sacrifices necessary. Here and in Chapters 2 and 3, I take up evidence that raises questions about our trajectory. First and foremost, we need to seriously interrogate the fundamental assumption underlying the commitment to finding and deploying cures: that doing so makes Americans healthier at reasonable cost.

Americans Aren't Healthier

A few years ago, I was a member of a committee for the Institute of Medicine, a component of the National Academies of Science.[5] The committee's job was to recommend ways to use resources to improve public health, and, after years of effort, we offered several. Our first recommendation was shocking to many. "The secretary of HHS should set national goals on life expectancy and per capita health expenditures that by 2030 bring the US to average levels among other countries," we said.[6] That's right; we recommended that the United States, the world's richest and strongest power, strive for average. How could that be?

We made our recommendation because, in spite of its enormous capabilities, the United States is below average when it comes to health outcomes per dollar spent. Way below average.

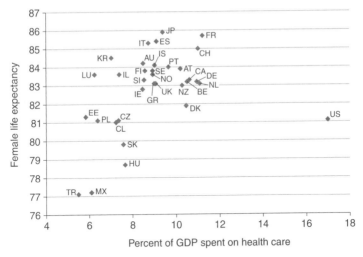

Figure 1.1. Relationship between percent of GDP spent on health care and female life expectancy in OECD countries. Missing life expectancy data estimates were imputed from prior year. Country abbreviations: AT: Austria; AU: Australia; BE: Belgium; CA: Canada; CH: Switzerland; CL: Chile; CZ: Czech Republic; DE: Germany; DK: Denmark; EE: Estonia; ES: Spain; FI: Finland; FR: France; GR: Greece; HU: Hungary; IE: Ireland; IL: Israel; IS: Iceland; IT: Italy; JP: Japan; KR: South Korea; LU: Luxembourg; MX: Mexico; NL: Netherlands; NO: Norway; NZ: New Zealand; PL: Poland; PT: Portugal; SE: Sweden; SI: Slovenia; SK: Slovakia; TR: Turkey; UK: United Kingdom; US: United States.

Data from the Organization of Economic Cooperation and Development (OECD) show that the United States is an extreme outlier in terms of expenditures (Figure 1.1). Per capita, the United Kingdom spends about $0.40 for each dollar spent in the United States; Belgium and Denmark spend about $0.50 for each dollar spent in the United States; Spain spends about $0.33.[7] Nevertheless, life expectancy is lower in the United States than in any of those countries. The populations of most member nations of the OECD are healthier than the population of the United States, according to this all-important measure.

Data from the US National Research Council backs up the OECD conclusions. The NRC considered current life expectancy for 50-year-old women between 1955 and 2010.[8] Current life expectancy is the median number of years of life remaining after a milestone age—as in, how many years can a woman expect to live after her fiftieth birthday? In 2016, that number was 33.15 years, according the US Social Security Administration, but the number varied considerably depending on demographic variables. In 1955 the United States was twelfth in the world on this indicator. By 2006 it had slipped to twenty-sixth, just below Malta. In a life-expectancy comparison of ten wealthy countries, US women were third out of ten in 1955 but ninth out of ten in 2006. Among the many countries with more rapid increases in life expectancy were Japan, France, and Spain, all of which spend far less on health care.

US life expectancy at birth also is not keeping pace. At the National Institutes of Health, we commissioned a National Academies study comparing US life expectancy with that of seventeen peer countries. The study was completed by a distinguished committee of physicians and public health scientists headed by Steven Woolf from Virginia Commonwealth University. Although US life expectancies are increasing, they found that the rate of increase lags behind that of our economic competitors. In 1980 US men and women were close to the center of the life-expectancy distribution among rich countries. By 2010 we had declined to last place for men and second-to-last place for women.[9] These studies also show that the United States experiences particularly high mortality rates from communicable and noncommunicable diseases. Among the seventeen countries, the United States had the second-highest mortality rate from noncommunicable diseases and the fourth highest from communicable diseases.

Perhaps the most surprising finding in the National Academies study concerns years of life lost prior to age 50 (Figure 1.2). The study committee considered international differences in the probability of celebrating a fiftieth birthday. The United States came in last on this indicator, with a loss rate twice that observed in Sweden. Although US men and women both fall at the bottom, the decline has been particularly acute among women. US men started at the low end of the distribution in 1980 and had worked their way to the bottom by 2006. US women also started near the bottom in 1980 and by 2006 were dramatic outliers, off the scale in relation to the comparison countries.

One of the major accomplishments of high-technology American medicine has been a decline in infant mortality—yet, even on that metric, the United States is in a shaky position. The good news is that, between 1999 and 2010, a 20 percent drop occurred in the number of babies born alive who died within the first year of life. The bad news is that the United States is still in last place among the seventeen countries in the international comparison. In nearly all countries, economically disadvantaged people have poorer childhood health outcomes; but high rates of poverty, especially among nonwhite Americans, aren't the whole explanation. When we control for socioeconomic factors by comparing only babies born to US and European non-Hispanic white women with a college education, the United States still has the highest infant mortality rate in the data set. The United States also has the second-highest rate of mothers giving birth to low-birth-weight babies in the seventeen-country comparison.

It is tempting to identify "the reason" for poor US performance in relation to peer countries. Alas, the committee found no single compelling explanation. What we can say with certainty is that the state of health in the United States is already worse than in peer countries, and we are losing ground.

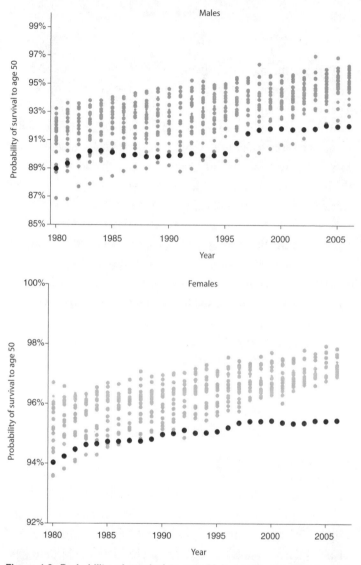

Figure 1.2. Probability of survival to age 50 in twenty-one high-income countries from 1980 to 2006, for males (top) and females (bottom). Black circles represent the United States. Gray circles represent other high-income countries: Australia, Austria, Belgium, Canada, Denmark, Finland, France, (West) Germany, Iceland, Ireland, Italy, Japan, Luxembourg, the Netherlands, New Zealand, Norway, Portugal, Spain, Sweden, Switzerland, and the United Kingdom.

American Medicine Costs Too Much

If good health were a commodity, Americans would easily be the world's healthiest people. Among competitor nations, we spend by far the most money on health care in absolute terms—$3.2 trillion per year—and as a percentage of GDP: 18 percent, compared with the OECD average of less than 11 percent. We are also the largest investors in biomedical research.[10]

It is important to recognize that we are not only getting less for our money than are the citizens of other nations; any time we spend, we also incur opportunity costs. If US health care spending were in line with that of our peers, we would save some $1.1 trillion per year, enough to fund all sorts of public goods such as education, infrastructure, industrial policy, social insurance, and defense. We could retire the national debt in about fifteen years.

Trends in state funding bear out the challenge of opportunity costs. Using data from public sources such as the General Accountability Office, I looked at local, state, and federal spending in five key areas between 1960 and 2016: health care, education, defense, non-health welfare programs, and transportation. In 1960, health care incurred the lowest cost among the five areas; in 2016, the highest. The largest decline was in defense spending, which was about 10 percent of GDP in 1960 and just over 4 percent in 2016. Education spending increased slightly between 1960 and 1980 but has remained largely unchanged since.

At the state level, it is easy to see how cost of health care has diverted resources from other pressing needs. In an article in *Foreign Affairs,* former Congressional Budget Office director Peter Orszag notes that, thanks in part to state outlays for Medicaid and other health programs, salaries for professors in public universities are now 15 to 20 percent lower than salaries in elite private universities.[11] California, my home state, has been hiking tuition throughout the University of California system, even as tax revenues rise, because the costs of MediCal, the state's Medicaid program, keep increasing. In 2017 MediCal spent $27 billion, 58 percent more than six years ago.[12] Historically, public undergraduate education has been the jewel in California's crown, but—in every state and at the federal level—all priorities are diminished so that we can fund the least efficient health care system in the developed world.

Few households can avoid the pinch. On average, American families now pay 23 percent of their income for health insurance premiums. In 1999 that figure was 11 percent. We are getting less in return, as deductibles and copayments increase. These costs also come out of wages and job opportunities. Faced with the high price of insurance, employers are less able to expand workforces and raise employees' pay.

No one would deny that Americans spend an unusually large amount on health care, or that the costs are rising, but not everyone believes the money is misspent. For instance, in a highly influential article proclaiming the value of expensive medical technologies, David Cutler and Mark McClellan argue that the increasing costs of treating heart attacks are worth paying. The authors, both high-powered economists who focus on public health, note that the cost for treating each case averaged $12,083 in 1984 and $21,714 in 1998, but new interventions produced, conservatively, a one-year increase in life expectancy, valued at about $70,000.[13] That is a net benefit of $60,000. NIH has cited this research while seeking funding increases from Congress.

Cutler, with Allison Rosen and Sandeep Vijan, made a more expansive case in the *New England Journal of Medicine* in

2006.[14] The article, "The Value of Medical Spending in the United States, 1960–2000," links improvements in life expectancy to medical spending. The authors measured the increase in spending during the time period and compared it with the number of additional years of life lived by various age cohorts. The best return on investment always follows treatments of younger people, and, after about 1970, the cost to save a life-year has gradually increased. Overall, however, return on investment is reasonable—supposing, as the authors do, that half of improvements in longevity result from medical care. Even for the oldest group in the most recent time period—when costs are highest—the price of an additional year of life is less than $150,000. A policy rule of thumb is that about $250,000 per life-year is reasonable. If my experiences in Washington are any indication, this article, too, has been influential, and mention of it arises frequently in congressional briefings.

But while analyses such as these have generated a lot of interest—Cutler and McClellan's article has been cited by nearly a thousand others—they do not persuade everyone. They are essentially expressions of status quo bias, assuming away the problems they are supposed to address. For instance, the threshold of $250,000 per life-year is not invented from whole cloth, but neither is it based on any law of nature. Policy experts decided on it, but no one is under any obligation to agree—to accept that the spending we now engage in is good for us because, on average, even old and sick people can have their lives extended a year for less than $250,000.

More important, the assumption that 50 percent of longevity increases are attributable to medical care is questionable, based on outdated and unreliable research. The two most important papers citing the estimate come from Lee Goldman and E. Francis Cook in 1984 and the IMPACT modeling group in 2004.[15] The

Goldman and Cook analysis focused on an observed decline in deaths from heart disease between 1968 and 1976. The authors estimated that about half of the decline was related to preventive care and the other half to improved treatment using coronary care units and advanced intervention methods. Their estimate was reasonable given the evidence available at the time, but key components of their calculation are not supported by current data. For instance, they believed that coronary care units could reduce by 88 percent mortality associated with heart attack complications. But more recent studies do not support this claim. For its part, the IMPACT model placed a great deal of faith in the coronary benefits of aspirin, arterial stents, coronary artery bypass surgery, and beta-blocker drugs. Enthusiasm for each of these interventions has waned in the past fifteen years. Other studies place the contribution of medical care to longevity at closer to 10 percent, with behavioral factors consistently accounting for a larger share of the gains than does treatment.[16]

Fortunately, we don't need to rely on models alone to figure out whether or to what extent our extremely costly health care is responsible for better health. Observational data show that care delivery and spending vary dramatically across geography, but with no discernible effect on health, suggesting that we should be suspect about the effect of care.

For example, a study of tube placements to treat ear infections among children in Maine and New Hampshire between 2007 and 2010 shows substantial variability in the rates of tube placement across similar communities. The variability persists after adjustment for age, sex, and type of insurer. Somehow, children in Berlin, New Hampshire, were more than four times as likely as children in Bangor, Maine, to have tubes. But there is no evidence that the former can hear better than the latter or are less likely to experience continuing ear pain.

Some of those children may have been born with the aid of a neonatal intensive care unit (NICU), another expensive medical tool the prevalence of which varies greatly, revealing mistaken health care priorities. There is no doubt that NICUs can provide dramatic benefits to premature and low-birth-weight infants. The problem is that we just have too many of them. The number of births per neonatologist ranges from 390 to 8,197, depending on location, and while the latter number is too high, the former is too low. In areas of the United States with the least NICU availability, survival rates of low-birth-weight babies are indeed poor. Beyond the lowest quintile, however, NICU availability makes little difference; high density of neonatologists is no better than moderate density.[17] On the whole, the United States oversupplies NICUs and undersupplies other intensive treatments for infants. In Spain, where there are many fewer NICUs per child but more resources for other kinds of care, infant mortality is lower than in the United States: 3.27 deaths per thousand live births versus 5.59.[18] It is worth investing, to a degree, in NICU services, but it doesn't take long for costs, and opportunity costs, to mount, even as we fail to achieve better public health.

Or consider Los Angeles and San Diego, just 120 miles apart. In 2006, Medicare spending averaged $11,639 per recipient in Los Angeles and $6,654 in San Diego for services offered during the last two years of life. Indeed, Los Angeles spent significantly more per person on every measure. However, evidence does not show that residents of Los Angeles are healthier than residents of San Diego. In fact, some evidence suggests that Los Angeles residents are worse off. For example, evidence from Medicare's hospitalcompare.gov consistently gives San Diego the edge on measures of patient satisfaction. The chances of dying within thirty days of major heart surgery are lower in San Diego than in Los Angeles. By 2012, the most recent year data are available, the spending gap had narrowed, but even then, per-recipient expenditures at the end of life in Los Angeles were 31 percent higher than in San Diego, according to the Dartmouth Atlas of Health Care.[19] Counting all Medicare recipients—not just those at the end of life—Angelinos cost 28 percent more in 2015 than San Diegans ($11,703 compared with $9,121) with no difference in health outcomes. The difference cannot be explained by variation in medical needs. Data on all indicators collected by the California Health Interview Survey show residents of the two counties place similar demands on the health care system and have similar health behaviors. For instance, rates of cigarette smoking and physical activity are comparable in the two regions.

The Dartmouth Atlas, breaking down health care use geographically, makes for stark reading. The maps show that the amount spent on health care and the number of services delivered differs greatly across geographic regions, with no relation to age, race, or sex distributions, or to the diagnostic profiles of given communities. For example, during the last six months of life, Medicare patients in New Jersey make an average of 13.5 physician visits, compared with 6.5 among similarly situated residents of Idaho. In Ridgewood, New Jersey, Medicare recipients used an average of $91,843 in health spending during the last six months of life, compared with $56,122 in Boise. Evaluations of the Dartmouth data find essentially no relationship between per capita spending and health outcomes across the United States. There does not appear to be a systematic relationship between per capita spending during the last two years of life and family ratings of satisfaction with care received. Perhaps unexpectedly, spending more did not buy more satisfaction; states with high spending tend to have lower patient satisfaction in the final two years of life.

Indeed, a variety of evidence links greater use of care with bad outcomes. Several analyses show that people are slightly more likely to die in communities where more acute hospital care is used. It could be the case that the populations of these communities are older, sicker, or poorer; however, the analyses controlled for age, sex, race, income, and variables related to illness and the need for care. But none of these factors explains the relationship, suggesting, again, that not only is more not better, it may be worse.[20]

Part of the reason for such wide variation in the rate and cost of care across locations is that medical needs are gauged subjectively. The Dartmouth group estimates that 80 percent of hospital patients are admitted with high-variation medical conditions—illnesses that tend to be diagnosed differently depending on the physician evaluating the patient. Such conditions include pneumonia, chronic obstructive pulmonary disease, gastroenteritis, and congestive heart failure. Because diagnosis is discretionary, hospital capacity influences the likelihood that a patient will be admitted. Studies show that the supply of beds explains more than half of the discrepancy in discharges for high-variation conditions.[21] In hospital-referral regions with fewer than 2.5 beds per 1,000 residents, the discharge rate for high-variation conditions was 145 per 1,000 residents. In regions with more than 4.5 beds per 1,000 residents, the rate was 219.8 discharges per 1,000 residents. Of course, discharges follow admissions.

The correlation between admissions and supply of beds suggests that, where care is available, it tends to be used—that oversupply is inducing high demand and not that supply is growing to keep up with demand that would otherwise be there. The Dartmouth studies use statistical models to adjust for the incidence of medical conditions in a given region, as well as for age, sex, and race, all of which are known to predict demand for health care. With these adjustments applied, it is clear that providers create demand for their services by diagnosing more illnesses. Similarly, we see that when new diagnostic technologies gain acceptance, new epidemics of disease appear.[22] This is an old problem: one of the earliest documented cases was described by J. A. Glover in 1938. Glover recorded the rates of tonsillectomy in the Hornsey school district of London. In 1928, 186 children in the district had their tonsils surgically removed. The following year, after the local doctor was replaced, the number of tonsillectomies fell to twelve.[23]

As the Dartmouth research and other studies show, the level of variation in health care services remains high today, thanks to supplier-induced demand and, probably, other factors. That variation doesn't seem to result in great differences in outcomes, suggesting that greater expenditures aren't buying us better health.

American Life Is Especially Risky

The cure narrative and the attending extraordinarily costly enterprise of biomedicine make some sense if we think of disease in a vacuum: when people are ill, they need treatment, so let's develop the best possible treatments. But while some illness "just happens," many health conditions have precursors in human practices. We know this from epidemiological studies demonstrating that nonbiological factors predict poor long-term health outcomes.[24] Another way to put it is that behavior and socioeconomic factors affect the risk of contracting disease.

Expensive cures do not address social and behavioral sources of morbidity.

Obesity is an important example of these social and behavioral sources of disease.[25] In 2014, 78.6 million American adults were obese, a rate of 34.9 percent. The OECD average is 17 percent. Genes play a role in incidence of obesity, but it is also heavily dependent on lifestyle choices and socioeconomic standing.[26] Conditions of labor, wealth, poverty, geography, and environmental quality can significantly affect obesity and resulting morbidity.[27] That the problem has mounted rapidly over the past thirty years speaks to its social and behavioral origins; genetic drift takes generations.[28]

Although biomedicine is somewhat successful in treating diabetes and other diseases associated with obesity, there is no biological cure for obesity itself—at least, not one that could be viable at the scale of tens of millions. And what success there is in treating obesity-related illness is ultimately a function of behavioral and social factors: responding effectively to chronic illness requires vigilance, time, and often money on the part of the afflicted. The need for treatment is of course very great: within the OECD, only Spaniards self-report a higher prevalence of diabetes than Americans. Other studies show that the United States has the second-highest diabetes rate in the OECD after Mexico.[29]

Another significant risk factor underlying adult disease is adolescent sexuality, the social and behavioral precursor par excellence. In the National Academies' international-comparison study, the United States had the highest rate of teen pregnancy, defined as pregnancy before the age of 16. The probability of teen pregnancy was 3.5 times higher in the United States than in peer countries, on average. This is important because giving birth prior to age 16 is a strong predictor of poor health outcomes later in life. Childbearing at an early age is not physiologically harmful. Teenage mothers are at lower risk for maternal death and ICU admissions in comparison to mothers in their thirties. The biggest risks accrue to mothers older than 35.[30] But teen pregnancy is associated with socioeconomic burdens that predispose young mothers to a trajectory that challenges their health. The United States also had the highest rates of syphilis, gonorrhea, and chlamydia contracted by people between the ages of 15 and 19 and the highest rate of HIV infection among those between the ages of 15 and 24. Appropriate education is far more successful than biomedical intervention in preventing incidence of these diseases.[31]

Anne Case and Angus Deaton, a Nobel Prize–winning economist, offer a particularly striking demonstration of the social and behavioral health risks Americans endure.[32] Using publicly available data for the years between 1989 and 2013, Case and Deaton studied death records from the United States, France, Germany, the United Kingdom, Canada, Australia, and Sweden. The researchers used other surveys to estimate ethnicity, educational status, and other demographic characteristics of the deceased populations. With this information in hand, they studied causes of mortality among various demographic groups between the ages of 45 and 55, years when the body is particularly sensitive to self-destructive behaviors and during which death is considered premature.

During the period studied, death rates among white non-Hispanics in this cohort declined in France, Germany, the United Kingdom, Canada, Australia, and Sweden. The United States was a different story. Death rates among American Hispanics fell, too, and at normal rates. But white non-Hispanic Americans have died at steadily higher rates since about 2000. Much of the increase was caused by behavioral factors such as suicide and poisoning by alcohol and opioid pain killers. A major biomedical driver of reduced life expectancy in this group is chronic liver disease, often a result of behavioral factors such as alcoholism, sharing needles, and unprotected sex.

The Case and Deaton study suggests that medical providers, usually in a sincere effort to relieve patients' suffering, are overprescribing opiates and thereby contributing to mortality among the people they serve. Some 15,000 Americans died from overdoses involving prescription opioids in 2015.[33] The problem extends well beyond overdoses, of course. The CDC estimates that, for each person who dies from an overdose of prescription painkillers, there are 825 nonmedical users. One hundred and thirty of these will become dependent; ten users will be treated for abuse, and thirty-two will be treated for overuse in the emergency room.

This is not just a social problem but also a health care problem. Our overreliance on biomedical treatment is killing thousands each year and ruining the lives of many more, and their families. And it is a peculiarly American problem: although some increase in deaths from prescription drug overdoses has been recorded in other countries, the United States is a dramatic outlier among its peers.[34] In 2015 there were 312 drug-related deaths per million Americans ages 15 to 64; in Portugal there were just 6; in France, 7; and in Italy, 8.[35]

One might contend that, even if social and behavioral risk factors can't be controlled medically, at least the health outcomes could thereby be mitigated. The solution, then, would be more medicine—more tests and more cures, available to more people. A study of 3,140 US counties or county equivalents between 1992 and 2006 suggests otherwise. The study finds that, in 42.8 percent of counties, female life expectancy decreased. The best predictors of premature mortality in these counties were living in the South, lower educational attainment, and higher smoking rates—not access to care.[36] Systematic studies indicate that these other social factors have considerably more impact on health outcomes than does accessibility of services.[37]

Getting to Average

What would Americans have to do to get to average in terms of health outcomes and expenditures?

Let's start with outcomes. American men, with current life expectancy of 75.64 years, are last among seventeen peer nations; we need to gain 2.37 years in order to reach the mean. US women, with current life expectancy of 80.78 years, are in sixteenth place. To be average, American women need to gain 2.17 years of life expectancy.

The question is, then, what can be done to make up these gaps. Should we turn to mammograms or weight loss? More medicine or social and behavioral change? The best data show that improving on social and behavioral risk factors is more worthwhile than investing in more medicine. Public health researchers Janice Wright and Milton Weinstein have developed a powerful model for estimating the gains in life expectancy that would result from either medical or socio-behavioral shifts. They find that individual choices of each kind are limited in their effects, but behavioral changes are, in most cases, most valuable.[38]

For example, Wright and Weinstein's model predicts that a woman who gets a mammogram every other year starting at age 50 increases her life expectancy by just 0.8 months. Pap smears are a bit more useful: a woman who gets a pap smear every three years starting at age 20 gains 3.1 months of life expectancy. More important is cigarette smoking: a 35-year-old man who quits smoking increases his life expectancy by about ten months, a woman by about eight months. That comes at a very low cost to the medical system—usually zero. A 35-year-old who cuts his or her weight from overweight to normal levels can expect an eight-month increase in life expectancy. Reducing moderately high cholesterol to the normal range, which could be achieved with or without medication, adds six months.

One sort of medical intervention that compares well is chemotherapy; for instance, patients with advanced small-cell cancer of the lung gain six to eight months from that intensive and costly treatment. This is in keeping with the strengths of American medicine: we are good at dealing with major diseases once they present themselves. A National Academy of Medicine committee finds the United States has lower-than-average rates of cancer and stroke mortality and better survival rates after 70 years old.[39] Americans are also better at controlling cardiovascular risk factors, including high blood pressure and cholesterol. What all this suggests is that, for society as a whole, the pursuit of average is served best through careful use of medicine and emphasis on social and behavioral change.

What about becoming average with respect to health care expenditures? According to a 2011 study in the *New England Journal of Medicine* by economist Victor Fuchs and physician Arnold Milstein, the average cost of medical care in Australia and Western Europe—places where overall health is better than in the United States—is about 10 percent of GDP.[40] The United States currently spends about 18 percent of GDP on health care ($3.2 trillion per year). If the United States were average in health care expenditures, we would save about $1.5 trillion per year. That is a savings equal to Canada's total 2015 spending on all goods and services, easily enough to pay for major needs at home such as infrastructure and better schools—or to retire our $13 trillion federal debt within a decade.

Conclusion

Cutting $1.5 trillion per year in health spending will not be easy, but one way to make progress toward that goal is to deemphasize biomedicine and refocus toward social and behavioral interventions. In Chapters 2 and 3, I dig more deeply into the evidence behind this claim and argue that we should be ready to take on the challenges of reform, even though they are considerable.

Failing to get to average means that more and more resources will be confiscated on behalf of a health care system that produces only mediocre outcomes. Preventable health conditions will continue to limit our workforce, making the economy less competitive. Reform always comes with difficulty, but, in the US case, maintaining the status quo is the riskiest strategy of all.

2

Research Promise and Practice

The world wars demonstrated vividly the military advantage to be gained from technology. Weapons, defenses, codebreaking, transportation, communication, medicine, feeding the troops: all the great historic challenges of war were met with technological advancement. But where World War I saw the maximization of an age-old style of combat, World War II was marked by fundamental transformations. Early electronic computers were just one area of dramatic innovation, categorically altering military planning and intelligence. And if anyone doubted that basic science had a place in technological progress, the atomic bomb convinced them otherwise.

In the decades after the war, the powers of science, engineering, government, and the armed forces would be enduringly yoked together in the military-industrial complex. As head of the Office of Scientific Research and Development (OSRD) during the war, Vannevar Bush was one of the founders of that complex. But while OSRD worked on behalf of the military, the research-and-development structure it fostered was widely applicable. Bush and others believed that peacetime problems, too, could be tackled through technological breakthroughs produced at the nexus of public money and basic science.

In July 1945, still in his capacity as OSRD director, Bush issued a report to President Harry S. Truman, "Science: The Endless Frontier." This seminal document laid out a grand vision for government support of basic science to benefit the nation. The best minds would find solutions to the most pressing challenges, highest among them the burden of disease. Bush's plan called for the transformation of American universities into research-intensive institutions heavily focused on biomedicine. The federal government would provide the necessary encouragement by directing large sums of money to the universities, to pay for both research and overhead.

But the government would not just toss cash at any scientist who came calling. Bush, Truman, and other scientific allies recognized that, if national priorities were to be met, federal agencies would need to set the direction of scientific work. And they would do so through a bureaucratic process of soliciting and reviewing grant proposals, making awards, and overseeing research studies. In biomedical research, the critical agency would be the National Institutes of Health (NIH).

Today NIH is the world's largest government funder of biomedical research, but its roots lie in a humble laboratory. The story begins in 1798, when Congress established the Marine Hospital Service to care for sick and disabled seamen. With increased immigration in the late nineteenth century, the service took on a public-health role, examining disembarking ship passengers for signs of infectious diseases such as cholera and yellow fever. Key to this effort was the service's Hygienic Laboratory, which operated out of a single room in New York City. By 1930 the laboratory, founded in 1887 to study bacteria, had grown considerably. That year it really took off, thanks to a $750,000 congressional appropriation to construct two new buildings. The same act of law reorganized the lab as the National Institute of Health (at that time singular).

NIH expanded dramatically after the war, as the so-called endless frontier of science appeared to stretch before the victorious Allies. Rolla Dyer, an early director, advocated for massive funding increases and helped establish what would become a hallmark of the organization: the combination of intramural research, executed in laboratories at the NIH campus, and extramural funding for universities and other research institutions. By 1948, NIH efforts had proliferated, with new research centers dedicated to cardiology, microbiology, and dentistry. The National Institute of Mental Health was founded a year later and diabetes and stroke institutes a year after that.

Financial support for biomedical research continued to grow almost exponentially until peaking in 1966, after which funding leveled off and then dipped amid concerns about the size of the federal budget. The Mansfield Amendment (reducing American troop deployment by 50 percent) further squeezed NIH by reducing Defense Department research outlays, some of which had been used to pay for medical studies. Faith in the problem-solving capacity of basic science is tenacious, however, and it would not be long before the government resumed its generosity. In 1971, NIH got a massive infusion of cash when President Nixon, following Vannevar Bush's example, declared a war on cancer. The National Cancer Act redirected money from a variety of scientific programs into NIH's National Cancer Institute, which remains the best-funded of its institutes.[1]

The good times have, for the most part, continued. Between 1999 and 2002, the total NIH budget nearly doubled. Another $2 billion boost came in 2016 under the 21st Century Cures Act, which directs investment toward personalized medicine, brain anatomy, stem cell research, and genomics. In fiscal year 2018 NIH got another 8.3 percent increase of $3 billion, bringing its budget to more than $37 billion. The House Appropriations subcommittee recommended that an additional $1.25 billion be added to the NIH budget for the 2019 fiscal year. However, the increase was targeted at specific biomedical programs, including Alzheimer's disease, the cancer moonshot, universal flu vaccines, and antibiotic resistant bacteria. None of the expansion was targeted at social, behavioral, and environmental determinants that account for most premature deaths in the United States. The same committee proposed a $663 million cut for the Centers for Disease Control and Prevention (CDC), the key agency tasked with keeping the public healthy.

American biomedical research comprises more than NIH, but NIH's enormous budget, talent pool, and influence on the work of private and university laboratories make it a defining force in the project of achieving better health. It is fair to say that the agency and its projects have few serious critics, admired as they are by Republicans and Democrats, university presidents, pharmaceutical CEOs, and nonprofit managers.

Alas, hype is not a source of health. For decades, we have been told that genomics and precision medicine—the cutting-edge research areas at NIH and the organizations whose goals it sets—will bring us personalized therapies to solve our own particular problems. We have been told that the drug-discovery process that begins with NIH-funded basic research generates astounding cures. Yet almost twenty years after the human genome was mapped, we await the first signs of useful genetic therapies. And the drug-delivery pipeline has become hopelessly clogged by flawed research, impractical studies, and corporate imperatives having little to do with patient needs.[2]

Meanwhile, the focus on genomics has only further committed us to biological determinism—the view that biology, genes in particular, determine health—and therefore the priorities of biomedical research and health care. We are stuck in a feedback loop wherein biomedical research begets additional faith in that research and crowds out other approaches to thinking about health. This despite the fact that the overwhelming majority of molecules patented as potential drugs—nearly 100 percent—are never used clinically.

For all our genius, our research process is beset by systemic flaws that undermine the quality and usefulness of scientific findings. In this chapter, I explore the failure of American biomedical research to deliver on its gigantic promises. We do need biomedical research, but not only that—which means we need to start questioning the hype.

Moonshot Medicine: Genomics and the Human Machine

The completion of the Human Genome Project is widely viewed as one of the most important milestones in the history of American biomedical research. The ambitious undertaking, which began in the early 1990s, was completed ahead of schedule, in a photo finish. On one side was Francis Collins and his NIH staff; on the other was Craig Venter, a biochemist and private entrepreneur, and his much smaller team. The race was tight and sometimes acrimonious.[3] In the end, the groups finished the task almost simultaneously and reported similar results. In June 2000, Collins and Venter joined President Clinton in a press conference to announce what they had done.

It was a heady moment. President Clinton assured listeners that the human genome project would "revolutionize the diagnosis, prevention, and treatment of most, if not all, human diseases." Collins predicted that genetic diagnosis was about five years away. Within ten years, he said, we could expect genetic therapies for major diseases. "Over the longer term, perhaps in another 15 or 20 years," Collins added, "you will see a complete transformation in therapeutic medicine."[4] The result of this transformation would be precision medicine, whereby physicians would use genetic information to tailor treatments to individuals, increasing the effectiveness of those treatments and reducing the incidence and severity of side effects.

Now we are about twenty years down the road, the "longer term" has passed, and Collins's prediction is a bust. As Timothy Caulfield writes in the *British Medical Journal,* almost none of the promise of the genomics revolution—gene therapy, detection of genetic precursors to disease, precision medicine—has been realized.[5] By 2012, more than 1,800 gene therapy trials were ongoing, but no cures had materialized. The largest benefits have been the development of drugs with better side-effect profiles and genetic testing to identify candidates for certain medicines.[6] We understand the genetic precursors of only a few serious diseases. Many people assume that we will find "the gene" for Alzheimer's disease, "the gene" for diabetes, or "the gene" for schizophrenia. But only a handful of serious diseases are associated with single-gene defects. Some forms of cystic fibrosis, Duchenne muscular dystrophy, and sickle cell anemia may be linked to simple abnormalities caused by specific genes. But most chronic illnesses, including diabetes, and most cancers are associated with hundreds or even thousands of genetic variants. Further, the multiple genetic defects do not act independently. They may interact in unknown ways. As a result, we still have little confidence in our ability to predict disease outcomes based on individuals' genomes.

The problem, at root, is that we expected too much from our knowledge of genes. For one thing, research carried out in the wake of the genome cataloging shows that genetic mutations are not as helpful in predicting disease as anticipated. For more than a dozen years, Nina Paynter and colleagues followed some 19,000 women, each possessing one or more of 101 different genetic mutations, to determine whether they developed heart disease or other associated conditions.[7] The researchers found that the presence of genetic mutations had little association with the development of heart disease, which means the mutations can't be used to make reliable predictions about heart disease outcomes. Genetic information provided scant incremental value over an old-fashioned interview and family history. The American Heart Association, after extensive screening, has identified only forty-five single nucleotide polymorphisms (SNPs) associated with coronary heart disease. On average, these genetic variations, which have been cherry-picked from the ten million candidates in the human genome, improve prediction of heart disease by about 5 percent. In contrast, simply asking about family history gives much more information. Having one parent who has experienced a heart attack increases risk by 67 percent. If the parent was less than age 50, the risk increases to 236 percent. If both parents had heart attacks by age 50, the risk goes to 656 percent in comparison to those whose parents did not have heart disease.[8]

Another much-ballyhooed approach to finding disease in the genes relies on particular mutations in individual nucleotide sequences. The idea is that, since we know that certain mutations can disrupt protein functioning, leading to disease, we should look for those mutations. If present, they might predispose a person to disease. Using modern computation, we can find these disease-associated mutations.

A study by Lisa Miosge and colleagues from Australian National University suggests that this approach does not work either. The researchers investigated mutations in twenty-three genes essential to the immune system.[9] In particular, they looked at deletions associated with conditions of illness. But they found that only 20 percent of the mutations predicted to be associated with observable diseases were actually associated with the conditions. Further, only about 15 percent of the deletions showed any discernible relationship to an observed disease or human characteristic. In other words, it is very difficult to differentiate between mutations that cause diseases and mutations that have little or no effect on the clinical expression of disease. This suggests that if we try to diagnose disease using genetic mutations as our guide, we will get the diagnosis wrong most of the time. In particular, genetic sequencing will produce many false positives.

Michael Joyner, a Mayo Clinic anesthesiologist, succinctly captured the fundamental challenges facing us when he coined the term "moonshot medicine." For most common diseases, hundreds of genetic risk variants with small effects have been identified, making it hard to develop a clear picture of who is really at risk for what. This was actually one of the major and unexpected findings of the Human Genome Project. In the 1990s and early 2000s, it was thought that a few genetic variants would be found to account for a lot of disease risk. But for widespread diseases like diabetes, heart disease, and most cancers, no clear genetic story has emerged for a vast majority of cases. Instead, says Joyner, "When higher-risk genetic variants are found, their predictive power is frequently dependent on environment, culture and behavior."[10] That is, if we want to unleash the promise of precision medicine, we need to better understand the complex relationships within the human body and between individuals and their social and physical worlds. In the United States, research into the first such group of relationships is now robust; the second, not so much.

Despite the failures of the past two decades, and what is increasingly recognized as the wrongheadedness of a gene-centered approach to precision medicine, support for the status quo remains high. In 2016 former president Obama announced a new Cancer Moonshot, which has received more than $2 billion in congressional funding. Much of that money is being directed to biomedical interventions leveraging genomics; very little is set aside for studies of, or prevention efforts related to, environment, culture, and behavior.

This is not to suggest that all boosters of precision medicine are blind to the important role of lifestyle in causing major disease. But their solution appears to be more genomics. They say that, even if genes alone don't determine disease outcomes, knowing genetic risks will motivate people to make healthy choices such as exercising more, smoking and drinking less, and using evidence-based medical services. As Obama declared in his 2015 State of the Union address, the genetic revolution provides "personalized information we need to keep ourselves and our families healthier."

There is little evidence for this claim. Virtually every systematic study on the subject finds that knowing one's genetic risk has only a small effect on one's health behavior.[11] This is understandable. We don't need genetic risk information to encourage behaviors that we already know are beneficial to health. Overwhelming evidence shows that just a few behaviors—such as engaging in physical activity and avoiding cigarette smoking—profoundly improve health outcomes, regardless of genetic risk factors.[12] For the most part, the public knows this, and anyone who knows their genetic risk factors probably realizes that lifestyle choices are important to their health, too. There is not much reason to expect that genetic risk information will motivate behavior changes that common sense and decades of heavily publicized research haven't.

So far, just about the only unambiguous beneficiaries of the genomics revolution are companies selling genetic tests to the public. The industry has flourished. One major player, 23andMe, offers a genetic test that has already been used by more than two million people, and market analysts predict the demand for genetic testing will continue to grow.[13] This despite the fact that at-home genetic testing products are notoriously unreliable. In 2013 the FDA noted that 23andMe's $99 saliva test—which was supposed to indicate risks for Alzheimer's disease, obesity, age-related eyesight loss, and breast cancer—was not "analytically or clinically validated." Long after it began marketing, 23andMe secured FDA approval for only one product. The FDA also found that the company OvaSure was marketing an unvalidated ovarian cancer screen likely to produce false positives that could lead to unnecessary surgeries. Another firm, SurePath, ran afoul of regulators for selling a human papilloma virus test of unknown sensitivity. Investigators also discovered that the KIF6 genotyping test, purported to predict heart disease and identify candidates for statin therapy, performed neither of these functions accurately. CARE Clinics' handy blood test, which is supposed to tell you if your child has autism spectrum disorder, doesn't work. Studies failed to link treatments for suspected autism to clinical benefits, suggesting that the patients identified as autistic in fact were not.[14] All of these tests attract more money into health care, yet they have no obvious benefits and may harm users by motivating bad decisions on the basis of false information.

Professional genetic testing can be more useful. It can help physicians determine whether women who have a certain type of breast cancer are candidates for the powerful drug trastuzumab (Herceptin).[15] However, the benefits may not be as powerful as we have been told. In 2018, the FDA permitted 23andMe the right to advertise their breast cancer screening products directly to consumers. The tests for BRCA1 and BRCA2 mutations identify women at increased lifetime risk for breast cancer. Although the advertisements are likely to be broadcast to all women via television, the mutations are actually quite rare. They occur almost exclusively in women of Ashkenazi Jewish decent. Even among these women, less than 2 percent have the high-risk mutations. For all other women, the chances of having BRCA1 or BRCA2 mutations are 0 percent to 0.1 percent. It may make some sense for women of eastern European Jewish heritage to be tested. For other women, spending the $199 and facing the potential anxiety may not be worth it.[16]

Genetic tests are also performed on some leukemia patients to determine whether they are candidates for treatment with imatinib mesylate (Gleevec).[17] And we know that the 3–5 percent of whites and 15–20 percent of Asians with the genetic polymorphism CYP2C19 need to avoid the blood thinner clopidogrel (Plavix).[18] But these are exceptions. To date, few therapies have been matched to genotypes, and a number of systematic reviews are pessimistic that many more such therapies will be found.[19] Further, we still have little evidence that the Human Genome Project spawned effective new medications. The two most widely cited examples, Gleevec and Herceptin, were patented and in testing by 1992—well before the completion of the genome study.

With all the bad press surrounding genetic tests, and studies consistently undercutting the promises of genomics, one might think that we would finally realize that our money hasn't been well spent. Yet the public can't seem to let go of the faith. It seems we are mostly genetic determinists, committed to the cure narrative and to the idea that the good functioning of the human machine is above all a product of biology. The appeal of genetic determinism is easy enough to discern: it offers the easy way out. Thwarting chronic disease with lifestyle improvements— an approach that medical studies and practitioners inevitably recommend—is a serious human challenge. Biological determinism offers the comforting possibility that we can be well without hard work and hard choices—or that these at least are pointless and so not worth the effort.

The theme of biology-as-destiny is prominent in the history of ideas about human heredity. That it remains pervasive today, however, may have more to do with public attitudes than with scientific theory. It is a measure of our faith in the biomedical approach that, where genetic links are proposed, skepticism seems to depart us. Thus, even as researchers have grown convinced that environmental factors play a pronounced role in health outcomes—and that, as recent discoveries in epigenetics demonstrate, gene expression itself is subject to environmental modification—popular writers are stuck in the old nature-versus-nurture mode.

In particular, news outlets make hay of supposedly strong relationships between genetics and complex, sometimes ill-advised, behaviors. Take the 2015 *New York Times* op-ed by the psychiatrist Richard K. Friedman, arguing that the sources of marital infidelity are genetic.[20] In this story, morals and social structures play a small role compared with genetically determined receptors for the hormones vasopressin and oxytocin, the latter believed to be associated with social bonding.[21] According to Friedman, those who strive for monogamy face "an uphill battle against their own biology."

But the evidence for biological influence over fidelity is thin. The argument is largely based on the observation that montane voles are sexually promiscuous and prairie voles monogamous. Supposedly this is because these rodent subspecies differ in their genetic receptor sites for vasopressin and oxytocin.[22] However, studies do not offer consistent support for this conclusion. It is true that the subspecies behave differently, but reliable evidence does not show that the genes affecting these receptors are responsible.[23]

Researchers have also linked genes and infidelity in humans directly, but so far unconvincingly. An influential 2008 study by Hasse Walum and colleagues claims as much, but it doesn't withstand scrutiny.[24] Walum's results purport to show that a particular allele—a genetic variant, in this case indexed as number 334—is strongly associated with pair bonding among men. In a survey, about 15 percent of men without allele 334 reported marital crisis or threat of divorce in the previous year, compared with 34 percent of those with two or more copies of the allele. But the study population is too small to allow a solid conclusion: that 34 percent amounts to just fourteen men. The researchers also ignored other possible associations, as they cherry-picked the ones they hoped to demonstrate. There is a strong possibility that the "relationship" here is attributable to chance.

Other studies further confound claims surrounding the behavioral effects of vasopressin and oxytocin genes. Research by Dorian Mitchem and colleagues using data from 7,378 Finnish twins found no association between extramarital mating and the variants of the oxytocin gene suggested by earlier studies.[25] The study does produce evidence of a relationship between genes and extramarital behavior, but it goes in new directions. In contrast to the Walum study, which suggested that effects for the vasopressin and oxytocin genes occur only in men, the Mitchem study observed similar effects in women but not in men. Further, the newer study did not find any association between extramarital mating and the specific variants of the oxytocin gene suggested by earlier studies. Overall, although producing interesting results, there are serious concerns about the replicability of earlier studies. In particular, there may have been a problem resulting from multiple comparisons. When studies use multiple outcome measures, about one in each twenty statistical tests is expected to be significant by chance alone. Thousands of tests can lead to hundreds of false positive results. Perhaps the most confusing aspect of the article is what the authors do not tell us: the number of people who had extramarital affairs. The article mentions only that very few of them did. At one point, it suggests that 9.8 percent of the men and 6.4 percent of the women admitted that they had had more than one sexual partner in the past year. However, only a fraction of these individuals provided genetic data. One has to assume that the conclusions are based on a very small number of individuals who had extramarital relationships. Perhaps this seems obvious, but critics sometimes let down their defenses when confronted with biological data they do not understand.

The possibility that behaviors are genetically determined or influenced is enticing for many reasons, and it can be a worthwhile area of research. But that doesn't mean we should believe bold claims such as Friedman's. So far, evidence for relationships between gene variants and complicated behaviors is tentative at best, and it is not getting stronger. That there continues to be such interest in threadbare findings of genetic-behavioral links shows just how deeply biological determinism is ingrained in our worldview, or perhaps how much we just wish it were so, absolving us of the hard work of healthful and prosocial behavior. It is no wonder, then, that after some twenty years waiting for the promised genetic medicine revolution, we are still holding out hope. And while we may eventually achieve breakthroughs in genetic therapies, one cannot help but wonder about all the other approaches to health we are ignoring in the course of this utopian quest.

Today's Moonshot: Precision Medicine

Most people with the same diagnosis get the same treatment. Even doses of medication tend to be fairly consistent across patients. Yet, we know that people are different and respond to treatments differently. Thus the current rage in biomedical research and practice: precision medicine.[26]

Precision medicine certainly is exciting in theory: the idea that we can use computational tools to tailor treatments precisely to individuals.[27] Databases will collect detailed information about people's health, medical records, and genomes, and investigators will sift through all of it using machine-learning algorithms and generate remarkably accurate personalized diagnoses.[28] Next, using programmed decision tools, computers will digest the relevant published medical literature to determine precisely what remedy is suited to a particular patient.[29] That system will use genetic information to recommend precise courses of treatment, for instance calculating a complex combination of several medications and their dosages, just right for one person and his particular illness. There will be no need to waste time and money testing treatments to see what works.

Clinical application of precision medicine is in an early phase, but health care providers are already advertising their skills in creating treatments that address the unique problems of individuals. Medical providers claim they can sequence your genome and identify the specific characteristics of your tumor in order to provide a cancer treatment precisely designed for you.[30]

It is essential that the buzz surrounding precision medicine not drown out the serious concerns it raises. For one thing, it assumes that genes tell us more about disease than they probably do. The pathology of most chronic illnesses is complex and unlikely to be easily explained by genetics.[31] For another, precision medicine risks a glut in diagnoses. The closer we look, the more likely we are to find some abnormality in any given person, and precision medicine promises the closest look we have ever taken. A system that scans hundreds of millions of data points associated with a single patient will probably find something that appears amiss. This will result in more treatment of patients without disease symptoms or with risk factors that may never lead to illness. The combination of overdiagnosis and overtreatment will further explode health care costs. We don't have much evidence of how precision medicine improves health outcomes, but we can safely assume that the incremental cost of such care will be large.

Precision medicine also faces important scientific challenges. Masses of information about individuals will be mined using the latest analytic methods. But millions of data points will be generated for each individual. Using traditional statistical methodologies, one significant observation will occur for each twenty statistical tests. The multiple comparisons problem remains one of the most important drivers of spurious results in science. The consequence of not attending to these problems will be overdiagnosis and overtreatment. Although precision medicine investigators are aware of this problem, a clear solution has not been forthcoming.

Finally, precision medicine may seriously undermine regulatory regimes we rely on to ensure the safety and effectiveness of medical care. Regulatory agencies such as the FDA rely on randomized clinical trials in which each person assigned a treatment condition gets the same care. This method does not apply well to studies in which subjects are assigned to treatment based on their unique individual characteristics. The samples available for a given study will necessarily be small, whereas measuring outcomes such as mortality usually requires thousands of study participants.

The proposed solution is that new products be evaluated on the basis of biomarkers rather than health outcomes. For instance, we will measure success by whether a precision treatment lowers patients' blood pressure, not by whether it serves to extend lives.[32] As I discuss in detail in Chapter 3, this is a central flaw of the biomedical approach. Improvement in biomarkers is often unrelated to the relevant clinical endpoint, which is longevity.

Before we add precision medicine to the physician's toolkit, we need to consider carefully its costs and whether the struggle to realize its potential is worth undertaking. From a scientific standpoint, it is an exhilarating problem. But its value to public health depends on how it compares to alternatives and whether it is able to address the sources of poor health. Precision medicine, like other clinical moonshots, consumes a lot of resources that could be directed toward social services, education, and other priorities whose benefits are more certain and more widely distributed.

Research Malpractice

In biomedicine, the cutting edge is often dull. Above I focused on genomics and precision medicine, but an additional chapter could be devoted to the stem cell revolution, which has been called in *Science* a "scientifically unsupportable exaggeration."[33] When ideas become entrenched, they grow resistant to new evidence.[34] In the sciences, this resistance is manifest in research priorities and in the research publication process itself. The result has been an ongoing parade of retracted studies. Scientists have learned to tell compelling stories even when the evidence doesn't back their case, and peer review, the principal barrier dividing science from speculation, isn't stopping them.

The British scientist Richard Horton suggests in the *Lancet* that about half of what is published in scientific journals is incorrect.[35] Some studies are based on small samples that are not representative of the populations for whom the results are generalized. Other studies that use large samples often report tiny experimental effects that could be meaningless for those seeking treatment. Rather than test a particular hypothesis with a clearly specified outcome, studies often assess many different outcome variables, increasing the likelihood that some positive findings occur by chance. Horton also points to frequent conflicts of interest compromising the integrity of findings. In the 2005 paper, "Why Most Published Research Findings Are False," the physician and statistician John Ioannidis argues that up to 80 percent of nonrandomized research studies and 25 percent of randomized trials produce results that cannot be replicated.[36]

It is rare that scientists report fake results, but improper findings do get published. One common avenue is known as publication bias: scientific journals tend to accept positive results— findings touted as evidence of some relationship or effect—and ignore evidence of nonrelationship and null effect. Journals want to publish exciting news. Null findings, commonly observed in research studies, are boring.[37] The consequence is that positive findings are rarely tempered by negative ones, leading to unwarranted exuberance.

Another problem is that published biomedical research is frequently useless. In a 2016 article, Ioannidis argues that most clinical research is of little clinical value.[38] He reviews several thousand medical research papers and concludes that the majority do not consider whether the context of data collection can be generalized to the scale of populations and whether the results are relevant to medical practice. For example, a study might subject participants to thirty days of hospitalization or continuous monitoring, options that few patients can afford or endure. And many studies test treatments far more expensive than alternatives that produce similar benefits. One wonders what good comes from a clinical study whose findings support only impractical therapeutic proposals.

The poor quality of publications reflects defects in the research itself. Indeed, some of the most common procedures in bio-medical research are subject to widespread errors. For instance, we have recently discovered that the cell lines biologists purchase and study in laboratories are frequently contaminated. A cell biologist may do an experiment using mouse cells, only to learn later that she had been studying guinea pig cells. In one case, investigators discovered that what they thought were ovarian cancer cells were actually breast cancer cells. According to current estimates, between 14 and 30 percent of cell lines used in laboratories are tainted or misidentified.[39] To its credit, the scientific community tried to respond to this serious problem in 2012 through the formation of the International Cell Line Authentication Committee. The committee now tracks more than four hundred known false cell lines.

In the case of contaminated and misidentified cell lines, the challenge lies in the experimental materials and so, presumably, could be met through auditing and better control of facilities and samples. It is harder, though, to correct our mistaken assumptions about how biology works—assumptions that lead to more bad and useless research. A core concern here is animal models, a backbone of basic research in biology. When scientists want to understand how human systems work, they look first to other mammalian systems on the assumption that what is true of one mammal will generalize to others, including humans. Thus we perform experiments using various rodents and other species in order to figure out how disease works in humans and which drugs might cure us.

But observations in one species rarely generalize in this way. This is so even among very similar animals, such as mice and rats. As a colleague from the National Institute on Aging told me during a recent conversation, "We have cured Alzheimer's disease at least three hundred times in mouse models, but so far failed to cure it in any humans." He was referring to a review by Jeffrey Cummings and colleagues documenting 221 consecutive failures in human Phase 3 randomized placebo-controlled trials of new medications to treat Alzheimer's disease.[40] The mathematician Norbert Wiener had it right when he quipped, "The best model of a cat is another cat—or preferably the same cat."[41]

The prevalence of animal models—especially mouse models—in scientific research cannot be overstated. An NIH analysis of 267,000 grant submissions received between 2008 and 2015 found that 190,329 (71 percent) either proposed mouse studies or incorporated mouse models in their rationale. Even though the number of new grants is declining, the number of grants proposing research using mouse models is increasing.[42]

The poor quality of research manifests in an epidemic of replicability failures. A flurry of recent articles in scholarly journals, such as *Science* and *Nature,* and popular outlets such as the *Economist,* has brought attention to the matter.[43] This replication problem is as large as the amount of spilled ink suggests. A 2015 analysis in *PLOS Biology* by Leonard Freedman, Iain Cockburn, and Timothy Simcoe finds that at least half of preclinical or basic science research studies cannot be replicated.

The authors estimate that about $28 billion are invested each year in irreproducible studies.[44]

The problem is not only widespread; it is also severe in individual cases, as differences between initial claims and second opinions can be enormous. For example, one analysis of a laboratory-based tumor treatment claimed 900 percent improvement in the survival of a mouse population. The replication study found improvement of only 30 percent.[45] In another case, a pharmaceutical company found it could not reproduce 65 percent of its own studies on potential drug targets—studies that had generated sixty-seven published papers. In 21 percent of these papers, published data were not consistent with the company's internal data. Another 7 percent of the articles had other inconsistences.[46] And when the Amyotrophic Lateral Sclerosis Therapy Development Institute tried to replicate nine promising studies of potential ALS treatments based on animal models, they got no positive results. This sort of finding, published in *Nature* in 2014, is as disappointing as it is common in animal-model research.[47]

Again, some elements of the reproducibility problem can be mitigated with better procedure—requiring the use of high-quality, verified reagents and cell lines, for instance. But we should be looking to more thoroughgoing improvements as well. For example, laboratory scientists need better training in statistics. And scientific practice has to be held to higher standards. In particular, clinical trial investigators should be required to pre-specify the primary outcome variables of their research and seek out the hypothesized relationship. Too much research takes advantage of chance relationships that crop up because investigators failed to prospectively declare the precise outcome they were looking for.

NIH announced in 2014 that it would take the problem of re-producibility more seriously. Director Collins and Principal Deputy Director Lawrence Tabak laid out in *Nature* new strate-gies for improving the replicability of preclinical research.[48] The 2018–2020 NIH budget authorization includes an admonition from Congress to stress the importance of experimental rigor and transparent reporting of research findings. It is too soon to say whether the new precautions and initiatives are producing a positive effect.

Where Are the Wonder Drugs?

Failures in the research process have a lot to do with the remark-able level of waste in the drug discovery, testing, and approval process. Imprecise science means that when researchers try to turn findings into therapies, they wind up with therapies, which cannot—and should not—sustain regulatory scrutiny.

Every year thousands of molecules are licensed in the hope that they will become blockbuster pharmaceutical products. Before they get there, though, they undergo three levels of rig-orous testing. Or, more accurately, some of them do—97.5 percent of new molecules and compounds never reach Phase 1, in which a drug is tested on a small group of people to determine the ap-propriate range of doses and identify unexpected side effects. Among those potential drugs that reach Phase 1, 2 percent go on to Phase 2, where they are given to larger populations and evaluated more extensively to assess efficacy and safety. Among the 10,000 compounds, only 5 reach Phase 3, at which point they are evaluated in very large populations, ideally from diverse racial and ethnic backgrounds.

Usually—56 percent of the time—drugs are denied approval because they are ineffective in everyday practice. Typically, this occurs when an early result cannot be replicated under the more stringent conditions of later trials. Although medical innovations are often introduced with great promise, their reported efficacy tends to decline.[49] One reason for this "voltage drop," as it is sometimes called, is that early trials are carefully controlled in ways that bias outcomes toward positive results. Later studies, involving more representative populations and use patterns, better simulate the messier experience of clinical practice.[50] The benefits of interventions under more realistic conditions are far less dramatic than the first results suggest.

Some drop-off between trials and real life is probably inevitable. Clinical trials test new treatments on carefully selected patients. In many cases participants are chosen because they are atypical. They have stable work schedules, adhere to their doctor's advice, and do not face many medical complications. It should not be a surprise that the tested treatments do not work as well on patients whose lives are complex and who face medical and social challenges. But that does not absolve the enterprise of biomedical research. At a minimum we should encourage more information on the value of interventions when they are deployed under real-world circumstances.

Pharmaceutical failures are not by any means the responsibility of scientists and regulators exclusively. We also have the drug industry to thank. Its priority is to make money, not to provide better health. Thus companies spend literally billions of dollars tweaking older, effective drugs in order to re-release them before patent monopolies run out.[51] With minor modifications to their products, firms can wrest drugs from the generic market, securing their bottom lines.

This perverse situation comes at great cost. While drug makers are reinventing the wheel, they are not pursuing real advances for patients. And their retread pharmaceuticals clog up the drug-delivery pipeline. It is no wonder that the lag between drug discovery and effective use in clinical situations averages seventeen years![52] Developing the basic science underlying a drug generally takes a few years. After this, pilot studies and proposals must be written, reviewed, rewritten, and resubmitted. Once a study is funded, it usually takes between three and five years to complete, and sometimes longer. Then the investigators need to write up results, which can take six months or more, especially in the case of complex collaborations. Next follows, typically, multiple cycles of peer review and revision. Once accepted, an article still may not appear in journals for more than a year, and it takes even longer for new work to gain the attention of other scientists in the field.[53]

We have known for some time that a serious problem exists with medical clinical trials. Most treatments are tested on highly selected participants and evaluated under circumstances that are quite different from usual clinical care. Testing treatments under these circumstances evaluates their efficacy, but efficacy trials don't measure the likelihood that the treatments will work in usual clinical care. For example, in some clinical trials, more than 95 percent of potential participants are excluded because they did not meet strict inclusion criteria, whereas in clinical practice, doctors are likely to treat a much wider range of patients.[54] The benefit of treatment under usual clinical circumstances is known as effectiveness. Defining the efficacy-effectiveness gap in health care is widely discussed, but most clinical guidelines remain loyal to data from efficacy trials. Large systematic reviews of the literature commonly identify important differences in outcomes by subgroup. For example, treatments for high blood pressure have been shown to reduce deaths in middle-aged people. But the same drugs apparently do not reduce deaths among older people.[55] Medications to lower cholesterol reduce heart attacks among people younger than age 60, but they have not been conclusively tested in people older than 75.[56] On the basis of studies of men, many drugs have been used for both men and women; only later did we learn that women respond differently.[57] Strict protocols common to clinical trial research that exclude classes of people also reduce the generalizability of the results.

We have yet to develop quantitative methods for estimating the difference between findings from artificial laboratory conditions (efficacy) and under real-world circumstances (effectiveness). But we do know that it is common for treatments shown to be efficacious in carefully controlled trials to lack efficacy when tested under real-world circumstances.[58]

After all the rejections and failures to replicate, and amid delays exacerbated by the imperatives of corporate profits, some new therapies do eventually come to market. But progress is becoming harder to achieve and more resource-intensive. As Anthony Bowen and Arturo Casadevall document in a 2015 study, "Increasing research investments, resulting in an increasing knowledge base, have not yielded comparative gains in certain health outcomes over the last five decades." In particular, they found that the amount of investment by the NIH between 1965 and 2014 correlated with the number of publications, but not with the number of new drugs. During the study interval, the number of new biomedical publications increased by 527 percent, the number of authors by 809 percent, and the NIH budget by a factor of greater than four. Yet over the course of those decades, the number of new molecular entities approved by the FDA rose by only 2.3 times.[59] In the meantime, as we have seen, Americans' life-expectancy gains have lagged behind Europeans' and, lately, have begun to reverse.

The Problem of Big Science

Historically, life science discoveries were usually made in small laboratories. For instance, the chemical structure of DNA was discovered by junior investigators with relatively few resources.[60] Circumstances are different now. The postwar research paradigm called for and funded coordinated efforts among large numbers of investigators and staff. After all, only with massive investment could science tackle an enemy as great as disease itself. The scale of military projects was successfully transferred to civilian life, a context in which so-called big science continues to thrive: today we have the $4.7 billion Human Genome Project, the billion-Euro Human Brain Project, and the $100 million NIH initiative Brain Research through Advancing Innovative Neurotechnologies (BRAIN).

Major programs such as these are capable of remarkable things. In physics, recent large-scale experiments calling on years of work from hundreds of scientists, engineers, technicians, and others have led to important breakthroughs such as the discoveries of gravitational waves and the Higgs boson. But in biology, the failures have been equally great. For all the capacity of big science, it is worth remembering that we have a lot to lose by putting all our eggs in one basket. Henry Markram's Human Brain Project is a case in point. Markram, a Swiss neuroscientist, has done brilliant work measuring electrical signals from freshly harvested rat neurons. His studies shed light on the process by which synapses—the structures linking neurons—are strengthened and weakened as a function of experience. Markram's findings helped us understand how brains learn.

In 2013, secure in his reputation, Markram launched an extremely ambitious project. His goal was to simulate the human brain's eighty-six billion neurons and hundred trillion synapses in order to research complex cognitive medical problems, including Alzheimer's disease. The idea was sufficiently exciting, and faith in Markram sufficiently great, that $1.3 billion was pledged by the European Union for the ten-year effort.[61] But some scientists balked. It seemed profoundly risky to bet all that money on the vision of a single scientist without any peer review of his project. In July 2014 more than eight hundred scientists signed an open letter challenging the venture. In response, Markram sought mediation to address critics' concerns. The mediators, a committee of twenty-seven scientists, issued a fifty-three-page report concluding that the project was in "disarray" and citing its extraordinary ambition as an impediment to success. EU member states were expected to contribute $570 million, but many have yet to make their payments.[62]

Another recent flop was the National Children's Study, which was approved during the Clinton administration. The study aimed to follow children from birth to age twenty-one in order to document environmental influences—physical, chemical, biological, and psychosocial—on young people's health and development.[63] The project eventually was funded for a dozen years at a cost of more than $1 billion, yet by the time it was cancelled in 2015, investigators were still fighting over the data-collection design.[64]

At this point, with about $450 billion invested in US scientific research every year, we have good reason to believe that diminishing returns have set in. A 2017 study by Stanford and

MIT economists agrees with Bowen and Casadevall's 2015 study, concluding that, while there are far more scientists today than in the past, their useful output has decreased on a per capita basis. To achieve the kind of scientific progress we enjoyed in the early 1970s takes twenty-five times as many researchers today. With respect to medical research in particular, the economists show that a significant increase in the number of publications and clinical trials has not been accompanied by proportionally greater life expectancy or drug approvals. Under the big science paradigm, they conclude, productivity is decreasing, and with it, return on scientific investment.[65]

Thomas Insel, who headed the National Institute of Mental Health for more than a dozen years, offered an interesting reflection on his vision as NIMH director. Insel was driven to find neurochemical and other quantifiable biomarkers for psychiatric disorders, and he openly expressed his reluctance to support behavioral research. But, later, he opined, "I spent 13 years at NIMH really pushing on the neuroscience and genetics of mental disorders, and when I look back on that I realize that while I think I succeeded at getting lots of really cool papers published by cool scientists at fairly large costs—I think $20 billion—I don't think we moved the needle in reducing suicide, reducing hospitalizations, improving recovery for the tens of millions of people who have mental illness." He concluded, "I hold myself accountable for that."[66]

Conclusion

In 2016 Congress gave NIH its first substantial budget increase in several years. In doing so, it doubled down on the status quo. A guidance letter attached to the appropriation reads, "The agreement urges the NIH director to continue the traditional focus on basic biomedical research." Placing their full faith in biomedicine, the appropriators explain, "The purpose of NIH basic research is to discover the nature and mechanisms of disease, and identify potentially therapeutic avenues likely to lead to its prevention and treatment. Without this early scientific investigation, future development of treatments and cures would be impossible." Congress specifically asked NIH to invest in precision medicine and to spend more on big science programs, including the BRAIN initiative, big-data projects, the Accelerating Medicines Partnership, the Human Microbiome Project, and the Cures Acceleration Network. No special requests were made for NIH to spend money researching social and behavioral factors affecting health.

In some ways, Congress's enthusiasm for basic science is heartening. We do need good biomedical research. But we also need more diverse research, encompassing more topics relevant to human health and attentive to the failures of existing methods. In Chapter 3, we take a closer look at a key reason why these methods often fail to benefit patients.

3

Mistaking the Meaning of Health

Getting a colonoscopy isn't anyone's idea of fun. For a week ahead of the procedure, patients have to discontinue blood thinners and some other medications. With a day to go, solid food, alcohol, and colored liquids are off-limits. Instead, patients take laxatives to ensure a "clean colon." At the clinic, anesthesia is administered—which itself requires recovery time—followed by the insertion of a long tube.

Most people feel the experience is worth it, though. Colon and rectal cancers make up the third leading cause of cancer deaths in the United States and are major causes of premature death overall. It seems obvious that there is much to gain from early detection. Thankfully, physicians and scientists are confident detection is in fact possible, through screenings. Colonoscopy is one of the few cancer screenings to receive an A rating from the US Preventive Services Task Force, a panel of the Department of Health and Human Services.

It turns out, though, that the medical community's convictions are not entirely justified. Studies do not show clearly that people who receive colonoscopies are less likely to die prematurely than are people screened using other methods. Indeed, screening in general has little effect on premature death. A study of 154,900 American adults screened using sigmoidoscopy (a procedure similar to colonoscopy, but performed with a relatively short tube) found that 2.9 percent of those screened died of colorectal cancers, compared with 3.9 percent of those not screened.[1] Other large studies have reached similar conclusions.[2] About 98 percent of adults screened will not die of colorectal cancers, compared with about 97 percent of those not screened.

More fundamentally, evidence does not show that colonoscopies extend lifespans. A Minnesota study found essentially no difference in mortality rates among patients randomly assigned to annual occult blood screening, biennial screening, or an unscreened control group. Each group encompassed more than 15,000 test subjects—large populations that reduce the likelihood of chance results. Over the eighteen-year follow-up period, 33.6 percent of the annual-screening group died from any cause, along with 33.4 percent of those screened every other year, and 33.6 percent of those in the control group.[3] Colorectal cancer screening may have a small effect on the likelihood of dying from colorectal cancer, but it doesn't have a discernible effect on premature death from all causes.

This is not an unusual story. Biomedical practice is afflicted by a shockingly basic deficit that fosters unwarranted faith in diagnostic tests and the treatments that follow: we measure the wrong things. In particular, we use various biomarkers, such as blood pressure and cholesterol level, to ascertain whether we are at risk for particular diseases. What we often fail to consider is whether interventions that improve biomarker scores actually lengthen life and improve its quality. In short, we do a great deal of health care without paying much attention to the essential components of health.

What Is Health?

Doctors get paid for what they do rather than for what they achieve. It is therefore likely that when a patient has serious side effects from medication, a provider will be rewarded in the

form of more office visits resulting in more revenue. More services are rendered, leading to overuse of medical care, excessive spending, and, in some cases, patient harm.[4]

What if we could reward the positive consequences of health
care rather than the number of services delivered—prioritize
value rather than volume?[5] As attractive as this sounds, it is not
easy to do. Prioritizing value over volume requires measuring
not just the medical process but also health outcomes. That, in
turn, requires a definition of health—something that has long
been, and may always be, a matter of debate. But although there
are many ways to think about health, two themes are essentially
universal. First, agreement is widespread that premature mortality is undesirable, so one aspect of health is the avoidance of
early death. Health encompasses more than life expectancy,
though, hence the second theme: quality of life. As an old saying
has it, "In the end, it's not the years in your life that count. It's
the life in your years."

Researchers have proposed several metrics to integrate life
expectancy and quality of life.[6] The goal is to settle on a defen-
sible method for measuring quality of life. A well-designed measure of life quality considers the disabling and diminishing
consequences of disease and disability. The best measures place
levels of wellness on a continuum anchored by 0.0 and 1.0 for
the highest level of wellness. In traditional survival analysis,
members of each birth cohort are scored as 1.0 if they are alive
and 0.0 if they are dead as they are followed each year. In
Quality-Adjusted Survival Analysis, quality of life can be used
to place each individual on the continuum between death and
perfect health. The outcomes are called quality-adjusted life
years (QALYs). The quality-of-life improvements gained from
treatment can also be calibrated. For instance, a disease that reduces quality of life by one-half, without reducing life expec-

tancy, will cut 0.5 QALYs per year. Both the advantages and disadvantages of health interventions can be measured in common QALY units. Various methods for measuring loss in quality of life resulting from illness or disability have been validated. Most measure how well people are functioning using questionnaires and account for the amount of time people experience a given state of health.[7]

Hypertension offers a useful lens for examining the trade-offs QALYs can measure, as well as the benefits of integrating mortality and quality-of-life information. Even though high blood pressure can shorten life, high blood pressure itself causes no symptoms. On the other hand, treatment for high blood pressure can cause symptoms and other undesirable side effects, while simultaneously extending lifespan. If treatments are evaluated only in terms of life expectancy, then their benefits will likely be overestimated because side effects and other costs will be ignored. A comprehensive measure accounts for all dimensions of health, providing a better overall estimate of costs and benefits of treatment.[8]

Refocusing health care on QALYs would be revolutionary. Doing so would help shift the health system away from delivering services and toward delivering results. But getting to that point in the United States demands that we discard faiths and assumptions critical to the current health care paradigm. Most concretely, it means paying health care providers for making their patients healthier instead of paying them for how many services they provide. Further, it would require doing away with our collective obsession with disease-specific mortality and instead thinking about whether interventions reduce mortality overall. If a patient dies prematurely due to cancer rather than due to heart disease, we may not have helped her. The goal is to measure benefits from the perspective of the patient. An important step in this direction will be accomplished by reducing our reliance on what are called surrogate markers.

Health Outcomes versus Surrogate Markers

By the numbers. That is how good doctors are supposed to practice. Your systolic blood pressure should be between 120 and 140 mmHg, and your fasting blood sugar should be less than 126 mg/dl. Good patients are supposed to think this way, too. The American Heart Association recommends that we all track our blood sugar, blood pressure, blood cholesterol, and body weight.[9]

But sometimes people with perfect numbers have heart attacks, and others with crummy scores escape illness and trauma. In spite of all the emphasis behind them, the numbers often tell us little. Consider that, according to the Framingham Heart Study, a 50-year-old man with high total cholesterol of 240 mg/dl, but no other risk factors for heart disease, has a 5.6 percent chance of suffering a heart attack in the next decade. If he brought his cholesterol level down to 195 mg/dl, he would reduce his risk to 3.7 percent. Stated another way, 94.4 percent of 50-year-old men with similarly high cholesterol will not have a heart attack in the next ten years, compared with 96.3 percent of 50-year-old men with normal cholesterol. Although cholesterol is a surrogate marker associated with heart attacks, significantly reducing one's cholesterol level only slightly changes the odds of being stricken (Figure 3.1).[10]

Surrogate markers tell us something about population-level risk but are not necessarily informative about individual health outcomes. Though the surrogate marker may be related to the clinical endpoint of interest, that is as much as we can say. So,

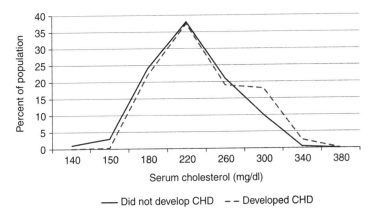

Figure 3.1. Serum cholesterol levels of men participating in the Framingham Heart Study aged 50 to 62 who later developed or did not develop coronary heart disease (CHD).

while heart disease and cholesterol are related, using cholesterol as a surrogate or substitute for heart disease can be misleading. This is true of other surrogate measures: for instance, the presence of tumors does not necessarily demonstrate elevated risk of death from cancer, nor do high blood-glucose levels always increase the risk of death related to diabetes. Improving one's numbers often leads to no beneficial health outcome.

Tackling All Causes of Death

Kurt Stange and Robert Ferrer make an important observation about the deficits of a treatment approach centered on surrogate markers and the particular diseases with which they are associated, which they call the "paradox of primary care": "Compared with specialty care or with systems dominated by specialty care," they write, "primary care is associated with the following: (1) apparently poorer quality care for individual diseases, yet

(2) similar functional health status at lower cost for people with chronic disease, and (3) better quality, better health, greater equity, and lower cost for whole people and populations."[11] How can it be that specialty care—the most advanced clinical manifestation of the biomedical paradigm—doesn't improve health?

One reason is that health outcomes are not the same as disease outcomes. Reducing the risk of suffering from one disease—something specialists are good at—doesn't mean that a person is healthy, in QALY terms. Yet, even though what matters to patients is overall health, biomedical research focuses on disease-specific mortality rather than all-cause mortality—whether an intervention reduces the chances of dying from a particular disease, not on whether it supports longevity as such.

The Physicians' Health Study, first reported in 1989, illustrates the problem. In this study, approximately 22,000 physicians were randomly assigned to take either 325 mg of aspirin or a placebo every other day. After participants had followed their assignments for an average of 4.8 years, the data indicated that significantly fewer physicians in the aspirin group had died of heart attacks: five aspirin takers versus eighteen in the placebo group.[12] This finding received extensive media coverage, inspiring an incalculable number of daily aspirin regimes.

But aspirin consumption did not in fact correlate with life-expectancy gains. Considering all causes of cardiovascular death—not just heart attack—there was no difference between the aspirin and placebo groups (Figure 3.2). Aspirin may have affected what was recorded on death certificates—fewer cases of acute myocardial infarction, aka heart attack—but the medication did not affect how long the study participants lived, on average.[13]

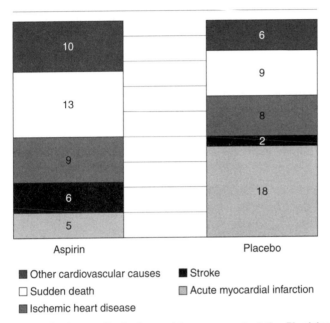

Figure 3.2. Total mortality in the aspirin component of the Physicians' Health Study. Overall, the number of physicians who died of heart diseases was identical in the aspirin and the placebo groups. Numbers in bar chart indicate numbers of deaths.

The use of surrogate markers to treat disease-specific mortality routinely produces this sort of outcome—helping reduce the chances that patients will die from a targeted illness—without affecting health. Consider the Action to Control Cardiovascular Risk in Diabetes (ACCORD) trial, which tested aggressive treatments of type 2 diabetes.[14] The aim of the trial was to reduce levels of glycosylated hemoglobin, a surrogate measure associated in type 2 diabetes patients with increased risk of heart attack and stroke. Researchers randomly assigned 10,251 type 2 diabetes patients to usual care or to an intensive-treatment condition. The intensive-treatment group received medical therapy

designed to lower glycosylated hemoglobin levels below
6 percent. The control group received standard care intended
to maintain glycosylated hemoglobin levels between 7 and
7.9 percent.

Looking exclusively at the surrogate measure, the treatment
appears successful (Figure 3.3). From the traditional linear perspective, the treatment was effective—it lowered blood sugar,
and high blood sugar is believed to cause diabetic complications
and early death. Those in the intensive-therapy group achieved
lower levels of glycosylated hemoglobin. However, 257 patients
in the intensive-therapy group died during follow-up, compared
with 203 patients in the standard-care group. Patients receiving
intensive therapy were also significantly more likely to develop
symptoms of hypoglycemia (low blood sugar). Ultimately, what
was good for one measure of diabetes control offered no benefit to overall health. Indeed, the risk of death from all causes
increased substantially.[15]

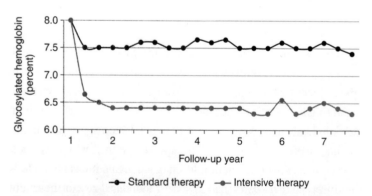

Figure 3.3. Differences in glycosylated hemoglobin for patients randomly
assigned to intensive therapy or standard therapy in the ACCORD trial. Intensive therapy clearly achieved the goal of better control of diabetes.

Another diabetes-drug trial, this one testing the FDA-approved drug sitagliptin, produced similar results. Developed by Merck and marketed under the trade name Januvia, sitagliptin also achieved better blood-sugar control than a placebo, as measured by patients' glycosylated hemoglobin. But, compared with patients receiving a placebo, sitagliptin patients experienced equal numbers of heart attacks, hospitalizations, and deaths from cardiovascular ailments.[16] On the basis of these and other studies, in 2018 the American College of Physicians (ACP) partially reversed its guidelines for the management of type 2 diabetes. Their new guidelines backed off aggressive management of blood glucose for all patients with type 2 diabetes. The ACP called for involving patients in discussions to personalize treatments in light of benefits and harms of drug treatments. Consideration should be given to the burden and cost of treatment in relation to how the treatment will increase health and life expectancy.[17]

Moving to the renal system, a trial with sufferers of chronic kidney disease turned out much like the ACCORD and sitagliptin studies. In the CREATE trial, scientists wanted to determine whether treatment with a drug that stimulates the kidney to secrete erythropoietin (EPO) would prevent anemia, which occurs when the red blood cells contain too little hemoglobin. Erythropoietin stimulates bone marrow to produce more red blood cells, a process known as erythropoiesis. Treatment with EPO had been shown under other conditions to increase hemoglobin levels, so it seemed a promising approach. To test their hypothesis, scientists randomly assigned low-hemoglobin adults with chronic kidney disease to either standard care or treatment with EPO. Members of the EPO group achieved normal hemoglobin levels within six months. But although the intervention did raise hemoglobin counts, it didn't lead to better health. Follow-up research found that those receiving EPO had higher red blood cell counts, but did not live longer or experience relief from symptoms. In fact, the EPO patients were more likely to end up with other symptoms and to be on dialysis.[18]

Diana Zuckerman and colleagues at the National Center for Health Research recently studied FDA approval of new cancer drugs and reached what is, by now, a familiar conclusion.[19] Among fifty-four newly licensed drugs, thirty-six were approved on the basis of promising surrogate markers—in most cases, tumor shrinkage. Yet follow-up data showed no evidence of improved life expectancy associated with half of the thirty-six drugs. In thirteen cases, manufacturers did not report survival data, suggesting that it may not exist; evidence of lifesaving effect is not something drug companies want to hide. Thus thirty-one of the thirty-six cancer drugs newly approved on the basis of surrogate markers do not, as far as anyone knows, increase life expectancy. Zuckerman's research also finds that only one of the eighteen drugs shown *not* to increase life expectancy was associated with improved quality of life. Two of the drugs reduced quality of life; one of these is still on the market, for $170,000 per person per year.

Let's look more closely at cholesterol and heart disease, where, in popular discourse, the connection between surrogate measures and health outcomes is especially strong. It is commonly understood that heart disease is prevented by reducing LDL cholesterol and increasing HDL cholesterol. To test the value of raising HDL, investigators in Europe undertook a large-scale project in which they randomly assigned 25,673 adults between the ages of 50 and 80 to take niacin, which is known to raise HDL cholesterol, or a placebo. The trial group also took a new medication to prevent a side effect of niacin consumption, flushing of the face, which tends to reduce compliance with niacin regimes. Participants in both groups were also given statin drugs, to lower their LDL cholesterol. The treatments did exactly what they were supposed to do in terms of cholesterol management: HDL levels rose, and LDL levels dropped. But changing cholesterol levels had no impact on death from all causes, including heart disease. There also was no evidence that modifying cholesterol levels delayed a first heart attack.[20]

A new class of cholesterol-lowering drugs, known as PCSK9 inhibitors, demonstrates the same disconnect between surrogate measures and all-cause mortality.[21] In a major industry-sponsored clinical trial, a forty-eight-week regimen of PCSK9 inhibitors reduced patients' LDL cholesterol to an average of 30 mg/dl, whereas a placebo group averaged a steady 90 mg/dl. Participants in both groups also took statin treatments, suggesting that these inhibitors are a better means of reducing LDL cholesterol. But while PCSK9 inhibitors brought LDL levels down, they didn't have much effect on disease. Among the treatment group, 5.9 percent of participants died of cardiovascular disease, heart attack, or stroke or experienced nonfatal heart attack or stroke. The rate in the comparison group was slightly higher, at 7.4 percent. Considering death from any cause, the groups were almost identical: 3.2 percent of the treatment group died during the 2.2 year evaluation period, versus 3.1 percent of the comparison group.

Some evidence shows that reforms of scientific-reporting policy can induce scientists to own up to a lack of patient-centered results such as improved all-cause mortality. In 2015, Veronica Irvin and I published an examination of all the large randomized clinical trials funded by the National Heart, Lung, and Blood Institute (NHLBI) during the last fifty years.[22] We were interested in whether the trials reported a significant benefit as a primary outcome variable. This is the variable that investigators typically use to justify their studies—the result they are looking for. To be included in the review, studies needed to indicate an important outcome, such as incidence of heart attacks and strokes and overall mortality. We found that, prior to 2000, positive results were relatively common, appearing in 57 percent (17 of 30) of published studies. After 2000, the success rate for large trials plunged to just 8 percent (2 among 25). Prior to 2000, twenty-four trials reported on all-cause mortality: five reported significant reductions in total mortality, eighteen a null result, and one reported significant harm. After 2000, no study showed a significant benefit in total mortality. All of the sudden, investigators were no longer so eager to make big claims about their findings. Why?

We don't know for sure, but, after controlling for other potential explanations, we speculated that the shift may have had something to do with the 1997 FDA Reauthorization Act, which required researchers to record their trial methods and specify primary outcome measures prior to data collection. Before 2000, the year the law was fully phased in, investigators could measure as many outcome variables as they liked and report only those that indicated statistically significant treatment benefits. But, with prospective declaration of the primary outcome variables, it became more difficult for investigators to selectively report some outcomes and exclude others. The new reporting standards may have initiated a move away from declaring death from any cause a primary study outcome.

Medical trials do at times demonstrate significant patient-centered benefits. NHLBI's recent Systolic Blood Pressure Intervention Trial (SPRINT) found that especially intensive treatment of high systolic blood pressure not only resulted in significantly fewer fatal and nonfatal cardiovascular events but also reduced death from any cause.[23] It was the first large NHLBI-sponsored prevention trial in more than twenty years to find reduction in all-cause mortality. And, the SPRINT trial had a big impact on policy. In 2017, the American Heart Association changed its guidelines and definitions of high blood pressure.[24] Just a few years before, another expert panel had recommended that, for people over 60, systolic blood pressures up to 150 mmHg were normal.[25] The new recommendation, based on the SPRINT trial, moved the goalpost. The new guidelines direct doctors to initiate treatment for anyone with a systolic blood pressure greater than 130 mmHg if they have more than a 10 percent risk of a heart attack or stroke in the next ten years. For people over 60, almost everyone is in that category. Only systolic blood pressures under 120 were considered normal. Those in the 120–130 mmHg range, by the new standards, are "elevated."

About a dozen years ago, Michael Ong and I analyzed the financial and health status benefits of these changing thresholds for treatment.[26] We discovered that the new definitions dramatically increase the number of people who will be defined as in need of treatment. Using data from the Health and Nutrition Examination Survey, we found that very few adults, only about 2 percent, could escape being classified into a disease or pre-disease category. The 2017 revised definition of high blood pressure immediately bumped the number of US adults with hypertension to 105.3 million from 74.1 million—an overnight increase of 31.2 million people. It also increased the number of people recommended to take antihypertensive medicines by 11 million.[27]

For people with high blood pressures, control can make a big difference. An 80- to 89-year-old woman who normalizes her diastolic blood pressure to 79 mmHg from a starting point of

110 mmHg would reduce her risk eightfold (from 0.0696 to 0.0081). This level of benefit is less likely for someone with initial blood pressure closer to normal. An 80- to 89-year-old woman who reduces DBP from 85 to 79 experiences a risk reduction for stroke from 0.0091 to 0.0081. In the SPRINT trial, 6 percent of participants who were given the intensive intervention had a heart attack or stroke during the four years of follow-up. In the control group, 8 percent had an event. So, the difference between those who did not have a heart attack or stroke was 92 percent versus 94 percent. Although the difference in deaths from any cause was statistically significant, by the end of the study 96.7 percent of the participants in the intensive treatment group remained alive in contrast to 95.6 percent of those in the control group. The absolute difference in survival is about 1.1 percent. But, intensive blood pressure treatment is not without risk. In the SPRINT trial, intensive intervention patients were 1.4 percent higher in episodes of low blood pressure, 1.1 percent higher in episodes of dizziness, and 1.8 percent higher in injuries to their kidneys.[28] Blood pressure treatments do save lives, just not as many as we have been promised.

Breast Cancer Screening: A Case in Point

Should women get regular mammograms? To many, the answer is a no-brainer: we all know screening enables early intervention, and early intervention saves lives. But is this true? In fact, a fair amount of evidence shows that breast cancer screening does not substantially affect life expectancy or quality of life.

I began studying the value of breast cancer screening in 1990, when I received a grant from the National Cancer Institute to assess methods for encouraging low-income Hispanic women to make use of mammography. At the time, the benefits of the diagnostic were relatively unchallenged, and it was widely believed that low rates of cancer screening among poor women contributed to that population's comparatively ill health.[29] So certain were medical experts of mammography's utility that the American Cancer Society used to run magazine ads featuring serious-looking women beneath the caption, "If you haven't had a mammogram you need more than your breasts examined."

In order to do a conscientious job, I wanted to learn everything I could about the value of mammography. I systematically reviewed all the large randomized clinical trials published before 1990 and found only minor benefits for women 50–64 years of age. Just one study showed benefits for women younger than 50, and it had serious methodological flaws.[30] In the last twenty years, several groups have reviewed the same literature and come to the same conclusion.[31]

As heterodox voices have gained in recognition and trust, breast cancer screening, particularly for younger and older women, has grown controversial. Medical organizations are now divided, with some strongly advocating mammography and others dismissing it. Table 3.1 summarizes just a few of the recommendations that came out between 2015 and 2018.

Major studies by the Pacific Northwest Evidence-Based Practice Center at Oregon Health and Sciences University, a Canadian task force, the Cochrane collaborative, a UK panel, the National Cancer Institute, and the US Preventive Services Task Force agree that women are 14–20 percent less likely to die of breast cancer if they are screened using mammography.[32] The results look very different, however, if we focus on death from any cause. No study to date shows a statistically significant association between mammography and reduced all-cause mortality, regardless of age group. Among all the studies, only

Table 3.1 **Summary of recent recommendations on breast cancer screening using mammography**

Group	Year	Recommendation
US Preventive Services Task Force (USPSTF)	2016	Mammography every other year, starting at age 50 and ending at age 70.
American Cancer Society (ACS)	2015	Annual mammography starting at age 45. After 55, mammography every other year. No age ceiling.
American Congress of Obstetricians and Gynecologists (ACOG)	2017	Annual mammography offered starting at age 40. Use shared decision-making for women older than 75 and for age to begin regular screening in individual women.
American College of Radiology (ACR)	2018	All women should be evaluated for breast cancer risk by age 30. Annual mammography for high genetic risk women starting at age 30; for asymptomatic women who are at average risk for breast cancer, annual mammography starting at age 40. No age ceiling.

Sources: USPSTS: https://www.uspreventiveservicestaskforce.org/Page/Document/RecommendationStatementFinal/breast-cancer-screening1; ACS: https://www.cancer.org/health-care-professionals/american-cancer-society-prevention-early-detection-guidelines/breast-cancer-screening-guidelines.html; ACOG: https://www.acog.org/About-ACOG/News-Room/News-Releases/2017/ACOG-Revises-Breast-Cancer-Screening-Guidance—ObGyns-Promote-Shared-Decision-Making; ACR: https://www.acr.org/Media-Center/ACR-News-Releases/2018/New-ACR-and-SBI-Breast-Cancer-Screening-Guidelines-Call-for-Significant-Changes-to-Screening-Process.

one obtained a statistically significant all-cause mortality result, but it was probably not one anybody expected. The Canadian study, a large and well-executed experiment, suggested that the death rate for women who were screened was higher rather than lower.[33]

A detailed review of observational data supports the notion that mammography is not very beneficial to health.[34] Some analyses have looked into breast cancer death rates across the United States in order to compare outcomes in regions with higher and lower rates of screening—as high as 89.7 percent and as low as 72.1 percent. At one time, the expectation was that cancer mortality would decline more rapidly in areas with greater per capita use of mammography services. But the data show similar declines in breast cancer mortality across regions.

Another sign that mammography is not responsible for significant reductions in mortality comes from a 2016 study of cancers that are routinely screened for, versus those not subject to routine screening.[35] The study tracks trends in mortality caused by fifteen different cancers, between 1969 and 2011. The investigators found that, while deaths from all cancers have been dropping since about 1990, the rate of decline is more rapid among cancers that were *not* ordinarily detected through screening tests.

A final word on mammography and all-cause mortality comes from the Swiss Medical Board, an impartial group of scientists and physicians who, in 2014, published a comprehensive review of literature from breast cancer screening trials.[36] On the basis of all the trials, the board estimated that, ten years after screening, between 951 and 952 of every thousand mammography recipients studied would still be alive. The board also estimated that 951 of every thousand women who did not receive mammography would be alive. Four out of a thousand screened women could expect to die of breast cancer, compared with five who were not screened. Among both groups, the board expects about forty-four out of a thousand to die from causes other than breast cancer in the ten-year period. The only reasonable conclusion is that, while mammography may have a small beneficial effect on breast cancer prevention, its contribution to life expectancy is virtually nil. On the basis of the analysis, the Swiss government gave up routine screening for breast cancer. A few years later, the minister of health released similar recommendations for France.[37]

If breast cancer screening provides little benefit with respect to all-cause mortality, it still comes with certain risks. In a 2014 study, Gilbert Welch and colleagues estimated that as many as two-thirds of 50-year-old women who receive yearly screening will experience at least one false alarm. Even a phone call announcing an unusual mammography finding can be extremely stressful.[38]

More importantly, false positives can result in unnecessary treatment. When a group of physicians and scientists supported by the American Cancer Society evaluated seven literature reviews, ten randomized clinical trials, seventy-two observational studies, and one applied statistical-modeling analysis, they found no clear evidence of greater life expectancy due to mammography, but they did find higher incidence of unnecessary biopsies. Among women who begin yearly screening at age 40, about 7 percent will have an unneeded biopsy within ten years. Cutting back to screening every other year reduces the rate of unnecessary biopsy to 4.8 percent.[39]

The most serious concern is that unnecessary treatments may result in illness or death. A faulty diagnosis based on false positives could lead to hazardous treatment with chemotherapy, radiation, or both. A range of studies documents the nasty consequences of chemotherapy on cognitive function, including memory and problem-solving ability.[40] Increasing evidence also indicates that radiation therapy increases the risk of heart problems, including death from heart disease. This risk sets in a few years after radiation exposure and lingers up to twenty years.[41]

A sober tally of the risks and benefits of breast cancer screening suggests we need to seriously rethink the frequency with which women are subjected to mammography. For many, this will be a hard recommendation to follow. But the evidence consistently shows that the roughly forty million mammograms American women receive each year are not extending their lives. That leaves the health value of mammography highly suspect.

Treat People—Not Diagnoses

A national survey conducted in 2004 found that 87 percent of American adults thought cancer screening was almost always a good idea. Nearly as many, 74 percent, believed that early detection saves lives. Almost 70 percent of respondents echoed the old American Cancer Society ads, telling poll-takers they considered a 55-year-old woman who did not get a mammogram to be irresponsible.[42]

It would seem, then, that a century of public health campaigns pushing early detection have made their mark.[43] Yet evidence that early detection results in better outcomes is limited.[44] Indeed, undiagnosed diseases are common and not necessarily harmful. The flip side of the coin is that high-sensitivity detection can give us information that scares us into unnecessary action. The question is always whether the harmful effects of treatment are worse than those of a disease that, while detectable, may not even have discernible impact on a person's health.

Consider that only about 3 percent of older men will die of prostate cancer and the same proportion of older women from breast cancer. However, breast cancer has been detected in 30 percent of older women and prostate cancer in 40 percent of older men who die from other causes.[45] Similarly, a study of 3,502 men and women over age 65 using advanced MRI technology found that 29 percent had evidence of mild undiagnosed strokes.[46] And although lung cancer screening leads to more diagnosis and treatment, clinical trials have shown that the course of the disease is likely to be the same regardless of whether patients receive screening.[47]

If screening doesn't affect outcomes, and one can survive undetected illness none the wiser, then the benefits of early detection are open to question, and the potential harms ought to be taken more seriously. For, the harder we look, the more likely we are to find what appear to be problems. The result will be that some patients end up with diagnoses and treatments that don't actually lead to better or longer lives. On this score, William C. Black and H. G. Welch make a useful distinction between disease and pseudodisease.[48] Pseudodisease is apparent illness that will not affect duration or quality of life. The remedy may have consequences, though, leaving the patient with new and more serious symptoms. What Black and Welch recognize—in contrast to much lay and even professional thinking about health—is that disease is not binary; it is not the case that people are either ill or well and therefore in need of treatment or not. In fact, most diseases are processes. Chronic diseases, in particular, call for different responses at different times, depending on how they affect quality of life.

Using information provided by patients, we can more accurately estimate quality-adjusted life expectancy for a population affected by a particular disease and thereby determine if that population is better off with or without screening and care.[49] Such an approach might seem shocking to the public, invested as we are in the early-detection narrative. It is therefore the task of physicians and scientists to bring nuance to our black-and-white paradigm and help patients understand that treating diagnoses is not the same as treating people.

Conclusion

At the moment, the United States is going in the wrong direction with respect to measurements of health outcomes. The 21st Century Cures Act enables rapid drug approvals by allowing pharmaceutical companies to use surrogate markers, rather than mortality and quality of life, as evidence of their products' benefits. A likely result is that drugs will get to market faster and, upon arrival, do less for our health.

The challenge, then, is to refocus the practice of medicine on patients. Rather than concern ourselves so narrowly with markers of potential disease, physicians and scientists should pay more attention to whether treatments actually help people live better and longer. Medical providers and institutions are starting to take important steps in this direction. For instance, the Patient-Centered Outcomes Research Institute, a public-private non-profit, was established in 2010 to fund studies of health care decision-making.[50] Their mission is, in part, to better understand which clinical practices actually produce relevant clinical outcomes, not just which are recommended for treating surrogate markers. Other organizations, including the American College of Physicians and the American Academy of Pediatrics, are beginning to refocus their missions on improving outcomes that are meaningful to patients and their families.[51]

4

Making Health Care Safe and Effective

In the year before he was felled by a stroke, President Franklin Delano Roosevelt had had his blood pressure checked repeatedly.[1] On March 27, 1944, it was 186/108. A few days later, April 1, it was 200/108. By November 18 it was measured at 210/112, and by February 1945, 260/150. On the day of his stroke, April 12, 1945, the president's blood pressure was 300/190.[2]

Roosevelt died from what may have been a preventable trauma. In the decades since, we have learned much about how strokes happen and how to avoid them by controlling blood pressure using drugs, lifestyle changes, and monitoring. Our growing capacity to avert and address the effects of strokes testifies to the power of an integrated approach to medicine. Improvements in basic science and therapeutic intervention are important here, but so are improvements in the behavior of both patients and the care-delivery system.

Yet, as detailed in earlier discussions in this book, the US health care system doesn't always work the way we would hope. More often, we act as though technical innovation and scientific advances can do everything for us. That's not to say that most of us have decided to oppose a more balanced approach to health, attentive to individual conduct, social circumstances, and the processes of research and care delivery. Rather, most of us don't even realize such an approach is worth trying, so convinced are we that the body is a machine whose creaky gears will be fixed through proper scientific understanding and medical engineering. This mechanistic orthodoxy is considerably to blame for our country's dismal combination of out-of-control spending and poor health care performance.

Beginning in this chapter, I turn to the benefits that can be achieved by looking beyond the mechanistic view and instead paying more attention to human factors. I begin with correctable errors and deficits that have accrued in care delivery as a result of systemic failure to rethink old ways. Many of our mistakes can be fixed without better medical knowledge or new medical interventions. Instead, simple tools such as checklists and quality metrics pay large dividends at a fraction of the cost of medical research and development. Although virtually nothing is invested in quality-improvement research—the federal Agency for Healthcare Research and Quality has a research-investigator-initiated grant budget of about $44 million, and their entire budget is less than 1 percent of that spent on biomedical research at NIH—efforts in this area have had considerable impact on the safety, efficiency, and effectiveness of certain health services. More quality improvement is needed, but gains so far should leave us confident in our ability to do better with what we already have—no moonshots required.

Health Care Is Hazardous

Over the past few decades, it has become increasingly clear that medical care is a source of considerable harm. One of the most influential studies on the subject, the Harvard Medical Practice Study, came out in 1991, and its findings have only been confirmed since.[3] The Harvard investigators randomly sampled records of 30,195 patients who had been hospitalized in New York and found that 1,133 (3.7 percent) suffered disabling injuries related to diagnosis and treatment. Specific sources of error included wrong diagnoses, surgical failures, errors in prescribing medication, and negligence on the part of care providers.[4]

The study provided the basis for a more detailed investigation conducted by the Institute of Medicine (IOM) of the National Academies of Science.[5] Published in 2000, "To Err Is Human: Building a Safer Health System" blamed between 44,000 and 98,000 hospital deaths each year on medical errors and estimated the total cost of such errors at nearly $76 billion annually. These findings placed medical errors as the third-leading cause of death in the United States. The list of hospital-acquired conditions associated with premature death is daunting: adverse drug events, catheter-induced urinary tract infections, bloodstream infections resulting from insertion of central lines in arteries, pressure ulcers, infections at the sites of surgical incisions, and on and on.

Critics decried perceived exaggerations in the IOM report, but follow-up studies show that in all likelihood the report underestimated the malign consequences of medical errors.[6] A recent analysis of studies published between 2008 and 2011 finds that preventable medical errors account for between 210,000 and 400,000 deaths nationwide each year.[7] The numbers come courtesy of quality improvement—impressive advances in record-keeping and data gathering that allow researchers to identify mistaken orders to stop necessary medications as well as laboratory results clearly indicating adverse patient reactions to treatment. The low estimate of 210,000 deaths per year still leaves medical errors as the third-leading cause of death in the United States behind heart disease and cancer. If the higher estimate is right, that means about five people die of complications from medical care for each one who dies of diabetes or Alzheimer's.

A 2015 IOM report, "Improving Diagnosis in Healthcare," focuses on one of the sources of preventable mistakes.[8] The authors define diagnostic error as "the failure to: (a) establish an accurate and timely explanation of the patient's health problem(s) or (b) communicate that explanation to the patient." They estimate conservatively that, in any given year, about 5 percent of those who see a health care provider in an outpatient setting receive an incorrect diagnosis. Another examination of decades of hospital records suggests that diagnostic errors contribute to one in ten patient deaths and are about twice as likely as other medical errors to be associated with patient death. Overall, between 6 and 17 percent of adverse events in hospitals result from diagnostic errors. Although diagnostic errors are relatively uncommon, people receive many diagnoses over the course of their lives, and, for most of us, at least one of those will be mistaken.

The 2015 IOM report identifies several strategies to improve diagnostic accuracy, including big-data approaches that take advantage of information technology to identify patterns in masses of clinical data. Big-data analysis is attractive but, as discussed in Chapter 2, can also be misleading, because many observed relationships occur by chance. For the most part, the report emphasizes the human element over the technological: our behavior and priorities are hurting us. The greatest challenge is to improve collaboration and communication among doctors, patients, and families.[9] The IOM report argues that clinicians get too little feedback about the acuity and accuracy of their diagnostic judgment and point out that little research is devoted to improving the diagnostic process and ensuring that choices of diagnoses are safe for patients.[10] Not only are diagnoses frequently incorrect, but physicians often have the flexibility to select a diagnosis for reasons unrelated to the best interests of patients. For example, some diagnoses may be favored because they involve tests and procedures that lead to higher physician payments. The selection of a diagnostic category has important implications for cost and patient outcome.

Errors have been building up in the health care system for many reasons. One is the fee-for-service model, which encourages providers to oversupply health care, leading to unnecessary or even harmful treatment. Another is that the results of basic biomedical research are poorly communicated to clinical investigators. For example, new treatments are often promoted on the basis of early-phase clinical studies or animal models, even when larger human studies question their effectiveness. Further down the line, the fruits of clinical research often may not be absorbed into medical practice.[11] Thus studies challenging the value of prostate and breast cancer screening have had only small effects on practice.[12] And, as we have seen, the clinical focus on surrogate markers and individual diseases results in a great deal of poor health care choices.

A major source of errors is the failure to do away with practices that outlive their usefulness. Physicians and medical researchers have adopted a term from management theory to describe this problem: exnovation. As the opposite of innovation, exnovation describes the tendency to neglect or obstruct improvements in what has been deemed the state of the art. A medical example is radical mastectomy. Theresa Montini and Ian Graham have documented the economic, professional, and social forces that maintained this practice long after evidence showed it to be ineffective.[13] Faith in the treatment was based on ideas about cancer biology advocated a century ago by the surgeon William Stewart Halstead. Halstead asserted that all tumors are destined to metastasize, which meant that the only way to save cancer patients was to extract their tumors and the tissue surrounding them. The radical mastectomy techniques he introduced in 1882 dominated breast cancer therapy for nearly a century.[14]

Several lines of evidence run counter to Halstead's position. Halstead believed that the radical mastectomy would cure cancers. But many women who underwent surgery had recurrences. Meanwhile, some studies show that some untreated tumors do not lead inexorably to death and may even resolve without treatment.[15] If tumors inevitably metastasize and radical mastectomy stops this progression, the extensive use of the procedure should have resulted in declining death rate from metastatic breast cancer. However, analysis of cancer registries shows that the incidence of cancer that was metastatic when first discovered has been stable at about 18 percent for decades.[16]

Radical mastectomies continued long after scientists demonstrated that simpler, less damaging procedures were just as good. In 1985, Bernard Fisher persuasively challenged the use of early, aggressive surgical therapy. He and his colleagues randomly assigned 1,843 women with breast cancers smaller than four centimeters to either have their entire breast removed or have the cancerous lump removed while sparing the rest of the breast. Those who had the lump removed also received radiation therapy. Five years later, 85 percent of the women who received lumpectomy were living, compared with 76 percent who had their entire breast removed.[17] Twenty years after treatment, the outcomes for the women in the two groups were equivalent.[18] Fisher's findings led to offering lumpectomy as the standard option in breast cancer treatment, but it took over a century to exnovate Halstead's ideas and procedures.

Failure to discontinue ineffective practices has consequences. Questionable but entrenched programs such as annual mammography and prostate screening consume money and time that could be put to better use. And if patients receive suboptimal or even detrimental care, their health may suffer. In the case of breast cancer treatment, thousands of women may have been exposed unnecessarily to a painful and disfiguring procedure. But although medical errors—and professional obstinacy—pose acute problems, we should not lose heart. Efforts already under way demonstrate that better practices are available to us. We know we can do better because we already are doing better, albeit not yet at the scale we need.

Quality Improvement Pays Off

In 2010, per the terms of the Affordable Care Act, the US Department of Health and Human Services (HHS) developed a National Quality Strategy, with the aim of making health care safer, more patient-centered, better coordinated, more evidence-based, and more affordable. A further goal was to ensure that treatments include behavioral practices. Fulfillment of these goals was assessed using 168 measures designed by HHS. For instance, the quality standards targeted risk factors for heart disease, including high blood pressure, smoking, and depression. To assess progress, researchers tracked blood-pressure numbers among patients diagnosed with hypertension, smoking rates among individuals age 13 and older, and the use of a standardized instrument to diagnose depression. Between 2010 and 2012, gains were made on 102 of the 168 measures. The greatest gains were in patient-centered measures such as self-rated health and satisfaction with care; improvements were seen in 85 percent of these indicators; 45 percent of patient-safety measures, twenty-four of forty-six effective-treatment measures, and eighteen of thirty-eight lifestyle measures also improved.

How was this accomplished? For the most part, through behavioral change, not medical interventions. In the early stages, HHS worked with practitioners to create logic models. The models identify steps necessary to advance safety. Based on the models, HHS and its partners created a number of programs and tools, such as the comprehensive unit-based safety program, aimed at reducing bloodstream infections associated with the insertion of central lines Another sought to prevent blood clots in veins. Yet another effort, Team Strategies and Tools to Enhance Performance and Patient Safety, enhances communication and teamwork skills among health care professionals. Finally, there was a concerted effort to develop surveys on patient-safety cultures and to track how organizations confronted safety challenges.

In December 2016, HHS estimated that these efforts to improve safety and effectiveness had prevented 125,000 deaths in hospitals and saved patients from 2.1 million hospital-acquired conditions between 2010 and 2014, representing a 17 percent drop in such ailments. The cost savings were estimated at $28 billion. Commenting on the project, American Hospital Association president Rick Pollock concluded, "While there is always more work to be done to improve patient safety, the collaborative efforts of hospitals and HHS have delivered great results."[19]

The HHS-led hospital-quality improvement project was inspired by the work of Peter Pronovost, a leading researcher in patient safety and health care quality.[20] Pronovost is one of the originators of systematic hospital checklists, a low-tech, human-centered approach to quality improvement that has garnered a great deal of interest and good press in recent years, including in writings by the physician and journalist Atul Gawande.[21] Pronovost developed checklists and other quality-control techniques to reduce the number of catheter-related bloodstream infections. Within three months of implementing Pronovost's system, hospitals saw a dramatic reduction in serious infections. The infection rate fell from 2.7 per 1,000 to zero, and the effect was maintained over eighteen months.[22] The American Hospital Association has continued to champion this method and spread it, leading to further declines in hospital-acquired infections.[23]

Quality improvement has been especially valuable in preventing deaths following high-risk heart attacks, such as ST elevation myocardial infarctions, or STEMIs. One of the most influential quality-improvement efforts has been the adoption of a standard "door-to-balloon" time, which refers to the period between a heart attack sufferer's arrival at the emergency room and eventual treatment by inserting a balloon into a clotted coronary artery. Once introduced via a catheter in the groin, the balloon is inflated to widen the artery, allowing blood to flow around the blockage to the heart muscle, providing necessary oxygen to the heart. An influential study published in 2000 showed that when door-to-balloon time is greater than two hours, patients are more than 50 percent more likely to die in the hospital, compared with those who receive prompt intervention.[24] Guidelines in place since 2001 recommend that door-to-balloon time be no more than ninety minutes. Today door-to-balloon time is an important metric of hospital quality and has been adopted as a core quality indicator by the Joint Commission on Accreditation of Healthcare Organizations. Worldwide, door-to-balloon time is getting faster, although in most countries there is still room for improvement.[25]

A related example concerns management of strokes, which also may require quick response times. In particular, patients experiencing thrombotic strokes, which result from blood clots in the brain that cut off the flow of blood to brain tissues, benefit from rapid administration of a medicine known as trans-plasminogen activator (tPA). A thrombotic stroke kills about two million brain cells every minute, but if tPA is administered promptly, chances of death and major disability are reduced.

However, one cannot give tPA to just any stroke sufferer. About 15 percent of strokes are hemorrhagic, resulting from bleeding inside the brain. Giving tPA in cases of hemorrhagic stroke can produce serious consequences, including death. So, before administering tPA, doctors have to be certain they have properly diagnosed the kind of stroke under way. This, however, costs precious time—and brain cells. Quality improvement can help ensure that patients are properly diagnosed and treated as quickly as possible.

Kaiser Permanente, the California-based health care giant, has been a pioneer in this regard. Their researchers studied the path of stroke patients from emergency room arrival to diagnosis and treatment and found a lot of wasted effort and time along the way. First, patients were taken to exam rooms to await a nurse. Then nurses would fetch a physician who in turn might summon a neurologist. All these steps precede confirmation that a stroke is occurring. Only thereafter would patients be taken to radiology for a CAT scan, which determines whether the stroke is thrombotic or hemorrhagic. At that point, candidates for tPA were weighed to determine the appropriate dose and sent elsewhere to receive the medication.

The Kaiser team recognized that many of the steps could be short-circuited, saving time. Under the new protocol, suspected stroke patients are never put in an exam room. When the ambulance arrives at the emergency room, a team swarms the patient, each member executing his or her role. Instead of moving the patient elsewhere to be weighed, a scale is placed under the patient while on the gurney. This way, the patient is already prepared for tPA administration, if a scan shows thrombotic stroke. The drug can be given immediately after confirmation of the diagnosis, while the patient still lies in the scanner. Overall, the new process can save up to thirty minutes saving as many as sixty million brain cells, which translates into better functioning after the stroke.[26]

Reaction time is critical when hospitals respond to emergencies, but quality improvement is also beneficial in the treatment of chronic illness. One example comes from an effort led by investigators at Cincinnati Children's Hospital, who brought together a national network of providers to develop best practices for care of children and adolescents suffering from Crohn's disease and ulcerative colitis, which typically are long-lasting and incurable. The project, ImproveCareNow, gathers and analyzes electronic health records to provide knowledge and decision support.[27]

Treatment of these illnesses is highly specialized and challenging for both physicians and families. Particularly in rural areas, patients may have little choice but to trust their welfare to physicians inexperienced in the management of Crohn's and colitis. It is therefore essential that researchers, physicians, patients, and patients' families have opportunities to share information and experiences and to learn from the wider population of patients and care providers. ImproveCareNow enables this sort of sharing, feedback, cooperation, and best-practices training among all stakeholders. The collaboration—involving seventeen specialized pediatric GI centers, 19,500 patients, and 575 physicians—has had a substantial positive result. When the effort began in April of 2007, only about half of the participating patients were in remission. With continual communication, information sharing, and the ongoing development of effective tools for managing Crohn's and colitis, the remission rate had reached 80 percent by July 2014.

Quality improvement has also led to better health among patients with chronic heart problems. In particular, blood-pressure control has gotten much better, which is critical to preventing untimely death. Unlike many surrogate markers that are unrelated to health outcome, blood-pressure control is consistently related to better health outcomes.[28] In population studies, a 13 percent reduction in blood pressure has been shown to reduce incidence of death from stroke by 21 percent.[29] Patients who take any of four generic blood-pressure-control medications and successfully manage cardiovascular risk factors such as cigarette smoking, high cholesterol, and diabetes reduce by 50 percent their chances of experiencing cardiovascular events and reduce their chances of premature death.[30] Thankfully, substantial evidence shows that almost everyone—regardless of their level of hypertension—can control their blood pressure.

The challenge is to get health care providers to screen for and adequately treat blood pressure and for patients to do their part by taking medications as prescribed. In other words, the difficulties in treating cardiovascular problems do not stem from a lack of knowledge; more than half a century ago, the Framingham heart study identified the factors associated with increased risk of heart attack.[31] Instead, there has been a failure to understand and use the information we have. A major problem is lack of awareness on the part of patients. Data from the National Health and Nutrition Examination Survey show that about a quarter of people with high blood pressure do not know they have the condition.[32] Among those aware they have high blood pressure, only about 60 percent are getting effective treatment. These numbers are also affected by demographics. Only about six in ten Hispanic survey respondents with observed high blood pressure knew they had the condition, and less than half were receiving effective treatment.[33]

What is to be done when medical knowledge and treatment methods are adequate to the problem, yet the problem persists? We don't need better research or care; we just need to ensure that we do a better job with the tools we have. Over the past ten years I have worked with the California Right Care Initiative to do precisely that—to disseminate better practices for the management of cardiovascular risk factors. Much of this project involves identifying high-performing providers, figuring out how they achieve their exemplary results, and sharing these practices with other providers.

It isn't hard to figure out which provider groups do best, as they report their performance on key indicators to the National Committee on Quality Assurance. The reports include information on the percentage of patients diagnosed with hypertension who manage to keep their blood pressure within a specified range. When we started tracking the data in 2007, Kaiser Permanente was the highest-performing provider on this score, with nearly three-fourths of their hypertension patients well-controlled. Not only was Kaiser doing better from the start, but they have continued to improve. By 2016 Kaiser had reached the 87 percent controlled mark.

Kaiser's approach upends traditional models of medical care. Instead of waiting for a person to make an appointment with her doctor, Kaiser is proactive. Kaiser's physicians measure blood pressure during every encounter. Patients diagnosed with hypertension hear from a Kaiser employee regularly to schedule evaluations by nurse practitioners or pharmacists, whose expertise in blood-pressure management often goes unused. Those few patients whose blood pressure can't be controlled by nurses and pharmacists alone are referred to a Kaiser internist and, if needed, a nephrologist or cardiologist. All patients with high blood pressure are entered into a structured protocol for managing treatment. They are tracked over time, with repeated assessments and adjustments to their treatment plans. Many other health plans use their own protocols to manage blood pressure, but Kaiser has achieved unusual success.[34] Kaiser initiates contact and relies on a range of providers, reducing barriers to effective care.

Kaiser also emphasizes the management of cardiovascular risk factors besides high blood pressure. In contrast to most medical groups, Kaiser has made tobacco control central to primary care. Data from the nationally representative Medical Expenditure Panel Survey (MEPS) show that only about half of smokers are advised to quit by their health care providers, and many providers don't even ask their patients if they smoke.[35] Kaiser's physicians regularly inquire about smoking and intervene when possible. Although rates of cigarette smoking are declining nationwide, including in California, the decline is sharper among Kaiser patients. Between 2002 and 2005, there was a 10 percent drop in smoking nationwide, a 7.5 percent drop in California, and, among Kaiser patents, a 25 percent drop. This despite the fact that, even in 2002, the smoking rate among Kaiser's covered population was lower than the national average. There is reason to believe that these efforts are paying off in better health. Although we do not have data on all-cause mortality, we do know that Kaiser patients are about 30 percent less likely to die of heart disease than are those with other insurance plans.

Thankfully, the practices that have worked for Kaiser and some other providers are not limited to them. The California Right Care Initiative has been successful in spreading quality improvement. When the project, which monitors blood-pressure-control protocols across all health plans in California, began in 2007, only about half of hypertension patients cared for by the state's medical groups had their blood pressure controlled. As of this writing, the figure is near 67 percent. The initiative has devoted particular attention to San Diego, where all the major medical groups are participating in a county-wide effort to improve blood-pressure management. Today, after seven years of Right Care involvement, rates of hospitalizations for heart attacks are down in San Diego County. The reduction is 16.5 percent greater than that of California as a whole. A recent paper in the *American Journal of Managed Care* estimates that the intensive quality-improvement effort in San Diego reduced health care costs there by $61 million.[36]

Conclusion

We know that providers who follow evidence-based protocols are more likely to achieve better outcomes for their patients. But our research infrastructure has devoted surprisingly little attention to the documentation of high-quality health care and to studies that systematically evaluate methods for improving the delivery of high-quality services. Investments in better care delivery might save hundreds of thousands of lives, but research on quality of care does not fit well in the biomedical paradigm, which encourages primarily basic science and the development of new drugs and medical technologies.

Still, we should not despair. Many services have already been shown to help patients live longer and better lives. Funding further research, and spreading the word about what already has been learned, is not easy. But at least we have many good ideas about how to improve the care we already know how to provide.

5

Social Determinants of Health

Long before anyone came up with the idea of a germ, people recognized that disease is in important respects a social phenomenon. One needs no understanding of microorganisms to recognize that epidemics are localized, tied to particular places and the people in them. Hence the separation of the sick from the well in the medieval leper colony and the quarantines during the black death. Hence too the obsolete miasma theory, which located the source of disease in surrounding air. Communicability and environmental embeddedness render disease an inherently public problem.

It might seem, though, that the microbiology revolution makes the issue moot. Ever since Sir John Snow traced London's 1854 Broad Street cholera outbreak to contaminated water, scientists have made extraordinary progress in isolating the vectors of communicable disease and eliminating them from the environment.[1] Cell biology made possible enormous advances in vaccination, cutting down infection rates dramatically. In 1900 influenza and tuberculosis accounted for nearly 25 percent of US deaths; by 2000, less than 4 percent. Today the big killers are noncommunicable, chronic illnesses. In 1900, heart disease accounted for about 6.2 percent of deaths; in 2000, more than 34 percent.[2]

This doesn't mean social factors are becoming irrelevant to health, however. It is enough to note that health outcomes are still powerfully tied to place. Average life expectancy differs on the other side of the globe and the other side of town. That's because locations are proxies for socioeconomic circumstance—

income, race, educational attainment, marital status, and so on. And correlations between longevity and social standing are very strong. Incidents such as the water crisis in Flint, Michigan, demonstrate starkly how public choices affect health, often along lines of class and race. Add it all together, and Asian women in Los Angeles can expect to live to 89, nineteen years older than the average black man there.[3]

As I discuss below, we have good reason to believe that social forces are not only associated with ill health but are also sources of it—sources that we can try to address. But the United States lags in social services spending. Elizabeth Bradley and Lauren Taylor note that the United States "spends less than 10 percent of its GDP on social services, while France, Sweden, Austria, Switzerland, Denmark, and Italy all spend about 20 percent of their GDP on social services."[4] This spending helps reduce poverty, improve school performance, mitigate the handicaps of discrimination, and promote healthful behaviors such as eating well, exercising, and refraining from smoking. Europe's consistent advantage over the United States in life expectancy suggests that social spending should be a major priority.

And yet, as we have seen, the tendency in the United States is to double down on fighting disease at the cellular level. Scientists lament that *too little* is spent on biomedical research.[5] A 2015 special issue of the *Journal of the American Medical Association* features five articles on the future of biomedical research, none of which contemplates social factors affecting health. Editorials from esteemed scientists such as NIH director Francis Collins and Robert Tjian of the Howard Hughes Medical Institute argue for more basic research, more clinical research—and not a word about research into social causes underlying the diseases they aim to remedy.

When research into social determinants of health is not ignored in high places, it may well be under assault. In the same year as the *JAMA* special issue, the US House of Representatives passed the America Competes Reauthorization Act of 2015, singling out National Science Foundation–supported research in behavioral and social sciences as "nonessential." The bill sponsor, Representative Lamar Smith of Texas, argued that while basic science research and technological innovation are presumptively in the national interest, other sorts of studies are not. The bill did not clearly define the nonessential disciplines, but the examples were almost exclusively in the behavioral and social sciences and included psychology, sociology, anthropology, and political science. The House also voted to eliminate the Agency for Healthcare Research and Quality, which studies the safety, effectiveness, and equity of health care.

The bill never made it into law, but the House majority's criticism speaks loudly about what they see as proper state objectives. Along with too many—though by no means all—scientists and medical providers, the government prefers to set aside social services and social science research and instead declare wars on disease. The biomedical paradigm is well-intentioned, but it is crowding out the kinds of effective health care interventions most urgently needed.

Poverty and Inequality Make Us Sick

Ample evidence shows a systematic relationship between health and social conditions such as wealth and poverty. A 2010 review of UK population-level data found that poverty is a better predictor of life expectancy than are traditional medical variables such as access to care, prevalence of early diagnoses, and rates of medical testing. Indeed, no factor examined in the study is as predictive as poverty. As the average income of given neighborhoods increases, so does average longevity.[6]

Washington, DC, provides a striking example of disparities even among neighbors, who live in similar environments and have access to the same hospitals. Paula Braveman and colleagues broke down the life expectancies of Washingtonians according to the nearest stop on the Metro, the city's subway system.[7] Residents of poorer areas around Union Station lived, on average, seven fewer years than did residents near Shady Grove station, in suburban Montgomery County. The distance between Metro Center and the wealthier East Falls Church is ten miles, nine stops, and eight more years of life expectancy. Between Foggy Bottom and higher-income Springfield-Franconia is a nine-year differential in life expectancy.

Perhaps the most striking example is the comparison between two neighboring zip codes in Philadelphia. These two neighborhoods, separated by just 4.1 miles, are decades apart in life expectancy (Figure 5.1). Babies born to families living near the Liberty Bell in zip code 19106 can expect to live to age 88, more than twenty years longer than those born in the neighboring north Philadelphia zip code 19132. Researchers at the Virginia Commonwealth University Center for Society and Health have identified at least six factors that account for these geographic disparities. Those in communities with lower life expectancies are more likely to have poorer access to quality education, unsafe or unhealthy housing, limited opportunities for safe exercise, closer proximity to sources of toxic agents and pollutants, less access to primary care doctors, unreliable or expensive public transit, and more exposure to residential segregation. Many of the factors are associated with differences in education and

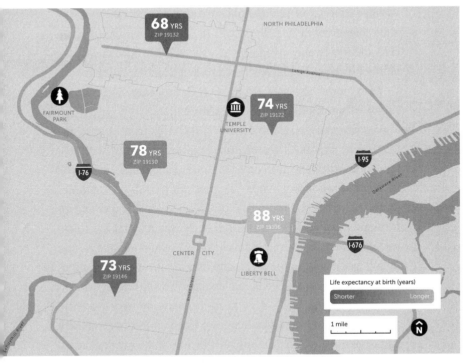

Figure 5.1. Life expectancies of individuals living in adjacent Philadelphia zip codes. The difference in life expectancy of those who live in zip code 19106 (88 years) is twenty years more than that of those who live in zip code 19132 (68 years), which is just five miles away.

income, and this clearly plays out in Philadelphia. In zip code 19106, 80 percent of the population hold a college degree and 41 percent have a graduate degree. In contrast, only 7.7 percent of zip code 19132 residents have a college degree, with 2.5 percent holding a graduate degree. Racial segregation is also apparent in the two neighborhoods. In 19106, there are nine white residents for each black resident. In 19132, there are forty-four black residents for each white resident.

Washington and Philadelphia are not unusual. In New Orleans, babies born near the lower-income French Quarter can expect to live twenty-five fewer years than those born in wealthy nearby Navarre. The researchers produced similar comparisons for neighborhoods in New Orleans, California's San Joaquin Valley, Minneapolis, and Kansas City, Missouri.

Another analysis, by epidemiologist Christopher Murray and colleagues, examines characteristics of communities with disparate life expectancies in order to isolate factors associated with greater and lesser longevity.[8] The most long-lived communities comprise residents primarily of East Asian background or northern, rural whites. The shortest life expectancies are found among low-income, rural whites in Appalachia and the South; Native Americans in the West; and blacks in rural communities and urban areas with high homicide rates. The differences across these groups are stark—15.4 years between the worst-off and best-off men and 12.8 years among women. Access to health care does not explain a significant portion of the discrepancies. Between 1982 and 2001, the rank ordering of life expectancies across the eight groups encompassed by the study changed little, suggesting that demographic gaps persist despite advances in medical science and technology.[9]

Perhaps the most persuasive study of the relationship between income and health outcomes comes from economists Raj Chetty, David Cutler, and their colleagues. They matched Social Security Administration death records with 1.4 billion tax returns reported to the IRS between 1999 and 2014 to explore associations between income and mortality.[10] Although the returns were anonymous, the data included information about the sex, race, ethnicity, and residence of taxpayers. It also supported estimates of insurance coverage and health care expenditures. The analysis, which included 4.1 million deceased men and 2.7 million deceased women, finds a clear association between higher income and longer life expectancy.

Women in the top 1 percent of the income distribution live 10.1 years longer than women in the bottom 1 percent. Among men, the difference is even greater, 14.6 years. Between 2001 and 2014, men in the top 5 percent of the income distribution gained 2.34 years of longevity compared with 0.32 years for men at the bottom 5 percent of the distribution. By the end of the study period, women in the top 5 percent enjoyed, on average, 2.91 more years of life, while the longevity of women in the bottom 5 percent was basically unchanged at plus or minus 0.04 years. Increases in life expectancy were not significantly associated with access to medical care, characteristics of the physical environment, or labor market conditions. However, people living in areas with more immigrants, college graduates, and government expenditures—areas that are, on the whole, wealthier—tended to live longer.

As these studies suggest, it is not just absolute income that correlates with health outcomes, but also income inequality. British epidemiologists Richard Wilkinson and Kate Pickett summed up this relationship in their 2009 book *The Spirit Level*.[11] Using an "index of health and social problems," which incorporated life expectancy as well as rates of mental illness, obesity, infant mortality, births to teenage mothers, homicide, imprisonment, educational attainment, distrust in others, and social mobility, Wilkinson and Pickett found an unmistakable correlation between income inequality and poor health and social consequences. The United States, the rich country with the highest level of income inequality, is an outlier, with by far the worst score on the index (Figure 5.2). Otherwise, scores on the index correlates almost perfectly with income inequality.

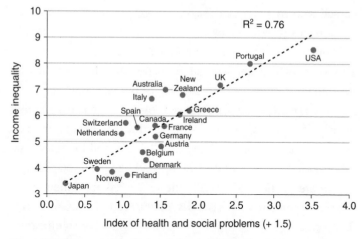

Figure 5.2. Income inequality in relation to index of health and social problems in selected countries. Income inequality is measured by the ratio of incomes among the richest 20 percent compared with the poorest 20 percent in each country. The index of health and social problems includes life expectancy, math and literacy, infant mortality, homicides, imprisonment rates, teenage births, level of trust, obesity, mental health, and social mobility. The index is represented in z-score units, with a constant of 1.5 added to eliminate negative values in the figure. Z-scores are defined as (individual score–average score)/standard deviation.

Although causation is hard to prove here, enough information is provided to establish it with high probability. As Wilkinson and Pickett show in a 2015 follow-up analysis, the relationship between health and income inequality is not only extremely strong, it is also consistent over time, and inequality always precedes poor health in time. A strong dose-response relationship is also found between inequality and health outcomes: for every incremental increase in inequality, there is a decrease in longevity. These findings, which satisfy requirements epidemiologists use to determine causality, should increase our confidence in the claim that income inequality is a source of ill health, not just a correlate. Wilkinson and Pickett also cite evidence showing inequality's effects on specific health outcomes. For example, they demonstrate that the consequences of leaving high cholesterol untreated are greater in countries with larger income disparities.

The argument is made still more plausible by data demonstrating that income gaps are associated with biological variables known to affect health outcomes. Wilkinson and Pickett review human and animal studies showing that social stress increases cortisol, which has long-term effects on memory and general health. In sum, Wilkinson and Pickett offer a persuasive argument that the correlation between inequality and reduced life expectancy is not spurious.[12]

The effects of inequality and poverty on health are particularly striking in the case of children, because deprivation in childhood carries forward throughout the life course. Not only does poverty potentially result in direct exposure to a variety of harms—such as criminality, effects of drug abuse, and environmental degradation—it also undermines development and is associated with increased long-term disease risk. A review of 201 studies from thirty-two European countries documented a consistent relationship between low family income and increased potential for diabetes, heart disease, and some cancers later in life.[13]

It is perhaps no wonder, then, that the American Academy of Pediatrics (AAP) has taken the lead among US medical societies in recognizing social determinants of health. Their 2016 report "Poverty and Child Health in the United States" draws on a substantial body of research showing the relationship between low family income and reduced birth weight, higher infant mortality, delayed language development, increased exposure to environmental hazards, and heightened risk of developing several chronic illnesses.[14]

AAP's focus on childhood poverty reflects the severity of the problem in the United States.[15] The US Census Bureau estimates that more than one in five Americans younger than eighteen lives in a household officially designated as poor.[16] Attacking childhood poverty is a significant challenge, although not insurmountable. Several government programs' interventions have worked.[17] Longitudinal studies suggest that income supplements cut the poverty rate nearly in half between 1967 and 2012. Without programs such as federal income tax credits and food stamps, about 31 percent of families would have been below the federal poverty level in 2012. With the programs, the observed level in 2012 was 16 percent.[18] The AAP recommends increasing these investments and supporting public programs to support employment of children from low-income families. The academy also has urged pediatricians to regularly assess patients' poverty status, so that they can be steered toward social service programs.

How Race Affects Health

Like wealth and poverty, race is systematically related to health outcomes. In the United States, non-Hispanic black men live an average of 7.3 fewer years than white men, and non-Hispanic black women about 5.9 fewer years than white women. Eighty-two percent of white women born today can expect to live to age 70. Among black men, that figure is just 54 percent.[19]

Why is it that blacks in the United States, both men and women, die from heart disease earlier than whites do?[20] Heart disease deaths are rare for all people younger than 45, but even in these age groups, black Americans die at a 50 percent higher rate than non-Hispanic whites.[21] Although race may be confounded with poverty and socioeconomic status, it explained differences in health outcome even with controls for socioeconomic status.[22]

Understanding the effects of race on health is fraught. It raises basic questions about what race is and whether race reflects meaningful genetic difference or is a constructed category applied to people for political reasons. Since the first US census in 1790, racial categories have changed at each ten-year interval when the census is repeated.[23] Evidence from studies of population genetics, the human genome, and physical anthropology show that humans classified in different races are highly genetically similar to one another.[24] And the history of race shows it to have highly elaborated juridical and social boundaries, whose biological meanings are constantly shifting. There is much good reason to believe that race is in our heads, not in our genes.

But we don't need to settle this debate. More important is to recognize that race, whatever it is, has long shaped the practice of medicine. "Race medicine" dominated the last few centuries.[25] Based on the belief that diseases behave differently in people classified as belonging to different races, it was promoted by prominent scientists whose opinions were used to justify black slavery. This despite the fact that, for centuries, medical research has consistently shown that diseases and treatments function equivalently across racial lines.[26] Racial stereotyping also has been shown to produce incorrect diagnoses that are based on stereotypes.[27]

The consequences of racial discrimination can also place people in risky environments. Because of discrimination, race can sort groups into different living circumstances, and in many cases selectively expose some people to greater environmental risk. Consider the water crisis in Flint, Michigan, which recently became perhaps the country's best-known example of adverse environmental effects on health—and the role that social factors can play in the suffering. A poor, minority-majority city, Flint was vulnerable to environmental and urban-planning failures that wealthier communities with well-funded public works are not likely to face.

The problems in Flint began in April 2014, when the city ceased purchasing treated water from the Detroit Water and Sewage Department. In an effort to save money, Flint decided that it would treat its own water, from the Flint River. But while Flint could do what was needed to make the water safe at the source, the city skimped on corrosion inhibitors—chemicals that prevent the water from corroding iron in lead pipes. Without inhibitors, the water caused lead to leach out of older pipes, leading to serious contamination.

What followed was a public health crisis. Lead exposure is toxic for people of any age, but it is particularly harmful for the developing brain.[28] In Flint, between 6,000 and 12,000 children were exposed to drinking water with high levels of lead. In 2013 about 2.5 percent of Flint's children had high levels of lead in their blood. By 2015, it was up to 5 percent.[29] In addition to causing problems with the developing brain, corrosive water can have other effects. The iron it releases creates a good environment for other bacteria, including *Legionella pneumophila*, which in turn can cause severe pneumonia. This is why the Flint water crisis was labeled as a probable cause of an outbreak of Legionnaires' disease that affected seventy-seven people in the county; ten of them died.[30]

Flint stood to save about $140 per day by forgoing corrosion inhibitors. In the end, the cost of fixing the damaged water-distribution system may be closer to $1.5 billion.[31] That doesn't include the long-term costs of caring for sick people, or the losses associated with lead poisoning. Lead poisoning is a tax on the future. It is especially damaging to the developing brain; children exposed to lead have an increased risk of learning disabilities, inattentiveness, and poor school performance.[32] In turn, these cognitive and learning problems are associated with social challenges and low income throughout life.[33] Each child adversely affected by lead exposure produces a continuing stream of costs to the health care, educational, and social service systems. Meanwhile, those kids are less likely to live up to their full potential. The problem of lead exposure in low-income black children is not limited to Flint. A study of more than a million blood samples from children in Chicago schools between 1995 and 2013 found significant racial disparities in lead exposure. The siting of low-cost housing near freeways and industrial sites is believed to be one source of the problem.[34]

Beyond exposure to pathogens, the experiences of adversity, abuse, and poverty can have an effect on metabolic, cardiovascular, and immune function.[35] Evidence suggests that greater exposure to psychological stressors, often a result of racial discrimination, can have significant long-term effects. One meta-analysis of 105 studies documented a consistent adverse effect of discrimination on a variety of health outcomes, including, in addition to physical health, strong adverse effects on mental functioning.[36]

Living Better Together

Studying social determinants of health can take a long time. Persuasive research requires years of surveys and tracking. Like

Wilkinson and Pickett, we need to know that relationships are robust over time, and that the arrow of causation points the right way.

The best studies of social factors underlying health therefore require a great deal of patience. One of the most useful began in Alameda County, California, in 1965 and finished up just a few years ago. The participants—6,928 adults living in the county—completed a series of questionnaires over the course of decades. Analyses demonstrated that the health habits of these adults were a major predictor of survival. For instance, individuals who smoked cigarettes, drank excessively, were overweight, spurned physical exercise, and got too little sleep were three times more likely to die of heart disease than those who engaged in none of these behaviors.[37]

The study also found that social life could have serious health consequences. In particular, investigators found a strong relationship between social support and health outcomes.[38] Those who were more socially connected, as measured by self-reported number of social contacts, had significantly greater longevity than those who were less connected.[39] These contacts include time spent with family and friends, as well as participation in community activities such as religious services and school-related events. When first reported in 1987, this finding surprised epidemiologists, but it has since been replicated in many different study populations and has remained robust in the Alameda population over the course of decades.[40] The English Longitudinal Study of Aging, which followed 6,500 men and women between 2004 and 2012, found that social isolation—measured through documentation of contacts with friends and family and through reported participation in civic organizations—was a significant predictor of survival.[41]

One of the forms of social connectedness easiest to study is also the most traditional: marriage. For reasons that are not entirely clear, being married and living with one's spouse improves one's health. With my colleague Rick Kronick, I assembled a data set that linked responses to the National Health Interview Survey to death records. Among the 67,000 survey-takers, 5,876 (8.77 percent) died before 1997. Controlling for age, race, income, and education, we found that those among the deceased population were significantly more likely to be unmarried or living without their spouses. Although the correlation was significant for unmarried people in general, it was strongest for those who had never married. In this population, no other variable was so strongly predictive of early death. Elevated risk of early death was greatest among men, although it was also observed in women.[42]

The association between partnership and longevity has been shown repeatedly, in diverse locations. A study of 9,333 British civil servants conducted between 1985 and 2009 found that marital status was a significant predictor of both cardiovascular and all-cause mortality. The age-adjusted mortality risk among men who were not married or cohabitating was 77 percent greater than that of married and cohabitating peers. Chance of death from cardiovascular disease was 169 percent higher. In this study, density of social networks was also a significant predictor of mortality, though the effect of marital status was greater. Again, women were similarly affected, but to a lesser degree than men.[43]

There are several possible explanations for the health benefits of marriage, partnership, and social support. It may be that friends and partners are particularly successful in urging healthful behavior and avoidance of harmful activities. The consistent finding that partnership and social contact generally afford men greater benefit than women—combined with other evidence indicating that women benefit from close connection with same-sex peers—is suggestive.[44] Unfortunately the data don't implicate any particular mechanisms underlying women's effect on their friends and partner's health, but we could speculate on a number of explanations that might be tested. It may be that women bring to their relationships greater knowledge of healthful behaviors; that women face greater social expectations regarding bodily fitness, which they then urge on male partners; that the benefits of partnership with women inspire men to treat themselves better in hopes of maintaining those benefits; or that the gendered system of household roles continues to ensure that women are more helpful than men in maintaining nutritious diets and clean, healthful home environments. Research is now beginning to isolate biological mechanisms that may explain the health hazards of social isolation more generally. Some evidence suggests that positive social interactions are associated with improved blood pressure and reduced body mass.[45] Another study finds that social isolation affects the expression of genes responsible for inflammation and down-regulates genes that produce antibodies necessary to fight infection. Specifically, socially isolated people were found to have deficiencies in monocytes—white blood cells produced in bone marrow, which play an important role in the early stages of fighting infection.[46]

Although not directly related to social isolation, a recent randomized, controlled study provides a tantalizing explanation of one means by which sturdy social networks can improve health. The study, which focused on a population of spouses and other family caregivers, demonstrated that a stress-management intervention reduced activation of the biological pathway that results in inflammation.[47]

Can Schooling Make You Healthier?

A rapidly accumulating body of evidence shows a strong relationship between education and life expectancy.[48] Within each tracked US ethnic group, among women and men, failure to obtain a high school degree is associated with the shortest average life expectancy. Longevity increases for those who finish high school and is greater still for college graduates.[49] Among white men, for example, the difference in life expectancy between those with less than a high school education and those with a college degree is about twelve years.[50] Those with master's degrees live longer than those with bachelor's degrees, and those with doctoral degrees longer than those with master's degrees.[51] In addition, poorly educated people report higher incidence of health-related disability than do more educated people.[52]

Using evidence from a database of about 33,000 black and white adults, I worked with colleagues at the University of Alabama, Birmingham, to test the apparent relationship between educational attainment and life expectancy.[53] We wanted to make sure other variables weren't responsible. We found that adjusting for income attenuated the relationship but left it intact. Adding demographic variables attenuated the relationship further but, again, did not eliminate it. The relationship also survives adjustment for medical and behavioral risk factors. On the whole, we were convinced that there is in fact a systematic relationship between educational attainment and life expectancy.

The American Cancer Society has found especially strong evidence of the education-longevity link. Using databases covering twenty-six US states, ACS researchers assessed all-cause death rates among individuals between the ages of 25 and 64, broken down by educational attainment. The researchers not only found a clear association between education and rates of early death, but they also found that the association is getting stronger. In 1993 men without high school diplomas were 2.5 times more likely to die prematurely than were men with college degrees. By 2007 the ratio had increased to 3.6:1. Among women the ratio increased from 1.9:1 in 1993 to 3:1 in 2007.[54]

The potential health benefit of education is far greater than that of nearly any medical intervention. Figure 5.3 illustrates the point. A pap smear every three years significantly reduces the chances of death from cervical and uterine cancer, but reducing the interval from three years to one year has essentially no benefit. Yearly mammography adds about one month of life expec-

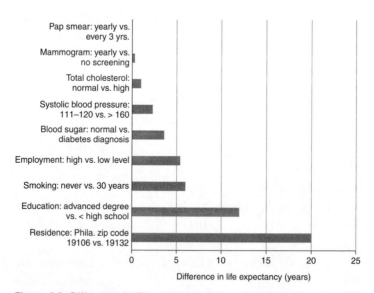

Figure 5.3. Difference in life expectancy for selected health and social factors. Common health care interventions have small effects in comparison with investments in social infrastructure.

tancy.[55] Bringing elevated LDL cholesterol down to normal adds about six months.[56] The difference in life expectancy between those with less than a high school education and those with an advanced degree is ten to twelve years.[57]

Education is more important to health than are other social effects. If we could eliminate homicide there would be about 12,000 fewer deaths in the United States per year. Eliminating fatalities from automobile collisions would reduce deaths by about 30,000 per year. Eliminating diabetes, itself powerfully influenced by social factors affecting diet and exercise, would reduce the number of deaths by about 80,000 per year. But ensuring that everyone gets a high school education could prevent an estimated 240,000 deaths per year.[58]

For the moment, there is no single, definitive explanation for the robust relationship between educational attainment and life expectancy, though there are many theories. Some studies suggest that schooling is associated with better health habits, perhaps as a result of continued exposure to pro-health messages in academic environments and of pressure to keep up with high-performing peers. For example, the probability of being a smoker declines with each year of education beyond high school.[59] Similar relationships have been observed with respect to physical exercise (better educated people get more of it), weight (better educated people are less likely to be overweight), and drinking (better educated people report fewer experiences of consuming five or more alcoholic beverages in a single day).[60] Some evidence also suggests that educational attainment can be reflected in the lengths of telomeres, nucleotide sequences that protect the end points of chromosomes. Shorter telomeres are associated with advanced age and shorter life expectancy, but it is believed that they can also result from biological responses to stress.[61] To the extent that lack of education is a cause of stress—perhaps because reduced earning power makes for financial and emotional hardship—there is a plausible biological foundation for education's health benefits.

Still, we have to accept a certain amount of uncertainty concerning the relationship between education and health. Like any social phenomenon, it can't be isolated in a lab. We can draw only from our observations, which vary with all sorts of contextual factors. For instance, Damon Clark and Heather Royer's natural experiment reveals a case in which more education did not correlate with increased longevity. They note that in 1947, England increased its legal school dropout age from age fourteen to fifteen. In 1972 the legal age changed again, to sixteen. In both cases, educational attainment improved, but no longevity gain was observable in the relevant student cohorts.[62]

This finding does not, however, refute the hypothesis that education benefits longevity. It may be that education has threshold effects. That is, just any increase in education won't ramify on individuals' longevity. Perhaps the difference between leaving school at fourteen, fifteen, or sixteen is negligible with respect to the biological factors affecting longevity. If in fact the fundamental issue is stress resulting from the career and financial handicaps of low educational attainment, then we shouldn't expect a large gap in the experiences of those who drop out at fourteen and sixteen. After all, the latter won't have much advantage over the former.

The problem of providing adequate, affordable education is perhaps as vexing as that of providing adequate, affordable health care. But to some extent they are amenable to the same policy solution: improving education can reduce the burden of illness.

Taking Social Factors Seriously

All the parties responsible for the American health care system—front-line care providers, insurers, scientists, charitable organizations, policy-makers—could do more to account for the social determinants of health. Small-scale change is already under way, an encouraging sign.

For doctors, nurses, and others who see patients, adopting what one might call a socially conscious approach is a simple matter of asking patients the right questions. Physicians have long understood the power of a patient history. Doctors inquire about prior health problems and injuries, previous experiences of medical care, and family history. Doctors also maintain medical records, providing meticulous documentation of case biology. But, until very recently, it was rare for health care providers to inquire about and record behavioral factors that might affect health. And systematic questioning about social and economic influences on health remains unusual. Learning more about socioeconomic circumstances may help individual patients have better health outcomes. And recording what is learned will help us substantiate the contributions of social factors to health, illness, and recovery.

The National Academy of Medicine has thrown its weight behind expanded medical records of this sort. An NAM committee recently recommended that health care providers make collection of "psychosocial vital signs" a routine practice.[63] These measures include race and ethnicity, tobacco use, alcohol use, and residential address. In addition, the committee points to substantial evidence that education, financial-resources strain, stress, depression, physical activity, social isolation, intimate-partner violence, and median income in the neighborhood of residence are relevant to health outcomes. Indeed, the committee argues that each of these factors is at least as important as the usual health information gathered during a medical history and physical examination.

As for philanthropic institutions, which have considerable sway in efforts to improve health, more should follow the example of the Robert Wood Johnson Foundation, which for decades been an influential voice in health issues. Recently, the foundation made an important move by transferring funds from some of its traditional medical initiatives into a program seeking to create a "culture of health"—"one in which good health and well-being flourish across geographic, demographic, and social sectors; fostering healthy equitable communities guides public and private decision making; and everyone has the opportunity to make choices that lead to healthy lifestyles."[64] Equal opportunity is a core component of the culture of health; RWJF has funded a $9.5 million effort to create better economic opportunities for middle-school-aged males from ethnically and racially disadvantaged groups.

RWJF has long recognized the importance of social determinants of health. That is why in 2007 it announced $500 million in grants aimed at reducing the rate of obesity. These are not grants for clinical care but for community organizations that work to get people exercising and controlling their diet. In 2000, the foundation launched the Cure Violence program, focused on reducing deaths from gun violence. Americans would be well served if other foundations concerned with health attended similarly to the social conditions that affect health outcomes.

Meanwhile, steps can be taken to encourage medical researchers to pay more attention to social determinants of health. Leadership from major funders and professional organizations will be essential in this regard. Researchers often have incentive to follow the priorities of these institutions, giving them great influence over the directions scientific study takes. For example, the American Psychological Association has increased focus on socioeconomic status by requiring all its journals to report income, occupation status, education level, social class, and related variables as they apply to all human study participants. Until recently, it was difficult to understand how research findings reflected social contexts, because this information was rarely disclosed in full.

Alongside medical institutions, policy-makers have a great deal of sway over research priorities. After all, they are responsible for much of the funding. So it is heartening that in February 2016, the Obama administration authorized the Centers for Medicare & Medicaid Services to give out $160 million in grants to community groups, health care providers, and others to screen patients for unmet housing and food needs and for experiences of interpersonal violence. One goal of the program was to assess whether addressing these problems would lower the cost of health care and improve health outcomes.[65] Although the Trump administration did not sustain the effort, researchers were able to develop useful data.

The United States could also do more with public money by funding social services directly. The US allocation between health care and social services expenditures is unusual within the OECD (Figure 5.4). Mexico, South Korea, and the United States are the only OECD countries that spend more on health care than on social services. Our total spending on the combination of medical care and other human services is about par for the course. Thus, deepening our commitment to social services—a commitment that seems to be paying off in our healthier peer states—doesn't require more cost, just different priorities.

Elizabeth Bradley and colleagues have shown that the international comparison extends to the US states as well. Using

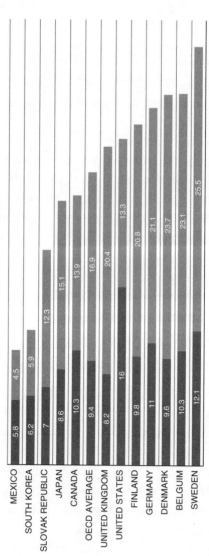

■ Health service ■ Social service

	Health service	Social service
MEXICO	5.8	4.5
SOUTH KOREA	6.2	5.9
SLOVAK REPUBLIC	7	12.3
JAPAN	8.6	15.1
CANADA	10.3	13.9
OECD AVERAGE	9.4	16.9
UNITED KINGDOM	8.2	20.4
UNITED STATES	16	13.3
FINLAND	9.8	20.8
GERMANY	11	21.1
DENMARK	9.6	23.7
BELGUIM	10.3	23.1
SWEDEN	12.1	25.5

Figure 5.4. Allocation of health services and other social service expenditures among selected OECD countries in 2005, as percent of GDP. Most wealthy countries spent, on average, $2 on non-health social services for each $1 spent on health care. The United States spent $0.55 for all nonmedical social services for each $1 spent on medical care. Total social spending is not exceptionally high in the United States compared with other wealthy countries, but the allocation between medical and nonmedical human capital spending is different.

2000–2009 data, she and her team calculated the rate of public spending on health and social services in each state and assessed how they performed on a variety of health measures. The researchers found that "states with a higher ratio of social to health spending (calculated as the sum of social service spending and public health spending divided by the sum of Medicare spending and Medicaid spending) had significantly better subsequent health outcomes for the following seven measures: adult obesity; asthma; mentally unhealthy days; days with activity limitations; and mortality rates for lung cancer, acute myocardial infarction, and type 2 diabetes."[66]

Conclusion

It is possible that spending more on health care, relative to social services, doesn't itself make people less healthy. It may be that poor outcomes per dollar reflect the need to spend more on medical care in places with more sick people, in which case the arrow of causality is reversed: high medical spending responds to high prevalence of health problems, not vice versa. But because the study has built-in time lags, measuring health outcomes one and two years after resources are spent, we can be fairly confident that funding decisions precede incidence of ill health. Although individual state circumstances will be a factor in any funding decisions, Bradley's research does suggest that policy-makers should be thinking hard about how to expand social services, even if doing so might result in diverting resources from health care.

Still, no matter how rigorously it is carried out, research on social determinants of health is likely to face skepticism. That makes sense: we usually cannot rely on traditional experimental methods such as randomized trials, so we need to be very careful about how we analyze social science data. But we also should be open to information those data can provide, rather than dismiss it as unscientific, "nonessential," or irrelevant to the health of the human-as-machine.

We are in the early stages of understanding social determinants of health. But it appears that the impact of many biological risk factors is dwarfed by the effects of social circumstances. We need to learn more about the effects of social stigma, the roles of education and income, and the consequences of social isolation. True, our most trusted research methods, such as the randomized clinical trial, are not well suited to determining causal relationships between social factors and health outcomes. That does not mean these factors can be ignored. We need creative new methodologies that will help us better understand health determinants and the interventions that may help extend life and improve the experience of it.

6

The Act of Well-Being

The top ten causes of death in the United States are associated with behavioral risk factors. Most of these killers are chronic diseases brought about by cigarette smoking, physical inactivity, poor nutrition, alcohol and drug abuse, self-destructive activity, and failure to comply with medical treatment. The causes of death and associated underlying roots are summarized in Table 6.1.

It stands to reason, then, that preventing and managing chronic diseases usually requires modification of behaviors, perhaps in combination with biomedical intervention. For instance, guidelines for managing high cholesterol and high blood pressure suggest lifestyle modification before the initiation of medication.[1] In practice, however, behavioral intervention remains uncommon in clinical medicine. A closer look at these behavioral problems makes clear how much is to be gained from these neglected interventions.

Deadly Behaviors

Drug Abuse
For the first time in many decades, US life expectancy is declining, thanks in good part to an epidemic of overdoses.[2] A major contributor to this worrisome trend is prescription opiates, which reduce physical pain but are also addictive. When patients get hooked, they may seek to continue treatment longer than necessary or turn to illegal and off-label options, such as heroin

Table 6.1 Behavioral risk factors for leading causes of death in the United States

Rank	Cause of death	Number of deaths	Behavioral risk factor
1	Heart disease	633,842	Physical inactivity, cigarette smoking, high-fat diet
2	Cancer	595,930	Physical inactivity, cigarette smoking, high-fat diet
3	Chronic lower respiratory diseases	155,041	Cigarette smoking
4	Accidents (unintentional injuries)	146,571	Alcohol and drug abuse
5	Stroke (cerebrovascular diseases)	140,323	Undetected and poorly managed high blood pressure, cigarette smoking
6	Alzheimer's disease	110,561	Head injury, smoking, poorly managed blood pressure. Other heart disease risks
7	Diabetes	79,535	Poor diet, physical inactivity
8	Influenza and pneumonia	57,062	Non-adherence with immunization schedules
9	Kidney disease	49,959	Diabetes associated with poor diet, physical inactivity
10	Intentional self-harm (suicide)	44,195	Self-destructive behavior, inability to access or take advantage of mental health services

Source: US Centers for Disease Control and Prevention. Health in the United States, 2016, table 19. Also available at https://www.cdc.gov /nchs/fastats/deaths.htm. Note data from 2015.

and fentanyl. The problem is clearly worsening: 2,888 deaths from drug overdoses were reported in 2004, 7,558 in 2014, and more than 64,000 in 2016.[3] Between 2001 and 2016 there was a 292 percent increase in the percentage of all deaths linked to opioids. In 2016, one in five deaths among 24- to 35-year-old adults was attributed to opioid use.[4] Social factors are at work, with drug deaths happening more often among those with lower income and less education.[5]

Coming to grips with the overdose epidemic requires a deep understanding of human behavior and better strategies for controlling pain and tolerating stress. One encouraging approach is to strategically wean patients off of opiate medications and teach them to manage pain using cognitive-behavioral therapy. Multidisciplinary teams have had success implementing these programs.[6]

Smoking

The year 2014 marked the fiftieth anniversary of the first Surgeon General's report on smoking and health. A report celebrating the anniversary summarized the remarkable accomplishments of tobacco-control programs. In 1964, 42.7 percent of American adults smoked cigarettes. University students smoked in class, commercial airlines allowed smoking onboard, and ashtrays were typically available on restaurant tables. By 2014 only 16.8 percent of Americans smoked tobacco, and the rate continues to fall. Smokers reduced their average daily cigarette consumption from twenty in 1965 to thirteen in 2014, and total per capita cigarette consumption has declined 60 percent during the same time period.[7] Figure 6.1 graphs the fall of cigarette use in relation to legal and social sanctions that are likely to have influenced the course.

As a result, the rate of lung cancer deaths has dropped, and the rate of emphysema deaths is beginning to fall as well. Deaths from heart disease, which peaked in the late 1960s, have declined at a rate paralleling the decline in cigarette use.[8] It is estimated that reduced smoking has saved six million people from premature death in the United States alone, accounting for at least one-third of life-expectancy gains during the twentieth century.

Surgeon General's reports have been hugely influential in reducing tobacco use, documenting thousands of studies showing that cigarette smoking can cause many serious diseases. Over time, the reports have touched on a wider range of tobacco's scourge-like health effects, making the warnings more persuasive.

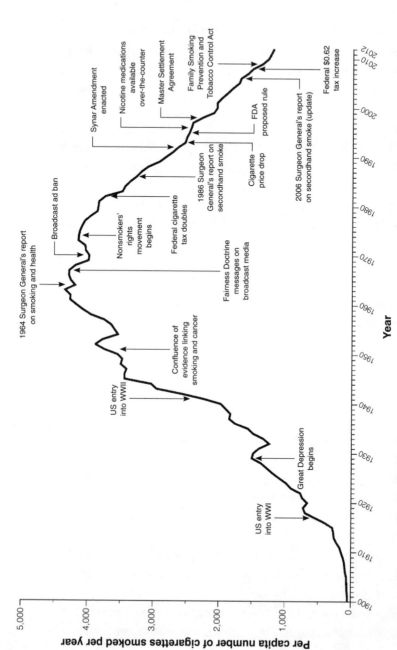

Figure 6.1. The rise and fall of cigarette smoking in the United States, 1900–2012. Figure shows adult per capita cigarette consumption in relation to major smoking and health events. Adults include those ≥ 18 years of age, as reported annually by the Census Bureau.

Initial reports concentrated on lung cancer, chronic obstructive pulmonary disease, and heart disease. More recent ones include evidence showing how smoking adversely affects virtually all physiologic systems, leading to rheumatoid arthritis, inflammatory illnesses, impaired immune function, birth defects among children born to pregnant smokers, and other significant problems.[9] Community groups, legislators, educators, and businesses organizations have seized on these findings to press for action, leading to bans on television advertising, restrictions on sales and marketing to children, state-level tobacco taxes, increasing federal taxes, prohibition of smoking in enclosed public spaces and some open ones, the end of smoking in bars and restaurants, and lawsuits resulting in the Master Settlement Agreement, which requires tobacco companies to pay more than $250 billion to support anti-tobacco efforts. In 2009 Congress and the White House enacted the US Tobacco Control Act, another important step, which gives the FDA greater authority to regulate tobacco products.[10]

Despite all these efforts, about 18 percent of US adults still use what historian of science Robert Proctor calls "a defective product" that is "unreasonably dangerous, killing half its long-term users," and "addictive by design."[11] The cigarette continues to be one of the few products that, when used as directed, can kill. Thus has cigarette smoking contributed to nearly twenty million premature deaths since the release of the first Surgeon General's report in 1964. Even with current restrictions on advertising, the 2014 Surgeon General's report suggests that, for each cigarette smoker who dies prematurely, about two new young smokers are recruited. Tobacco marketers spend approximately $1 million every hour to recruit new smokers.[12] US tobacco sellers have also expanded their influence campaigns overseas to make up for losses at home.

Prabhat Jha and Richard Peto report that, globally, about 50 percent of men and 10 percent of women are initiating a smoking habit during their lifetimes. Most smokers will not quit early; if current trends continue, worldwide deaths attributable to tobacco smoking will rise from about five million in 2010 to more than ten million in the next few decades. In most countries, the difference in life expectancy between current smokers and those who have never smoked is at least a decade.[13] Jha and Peto's analysis shows more adverse effects for cigarette smoking than did previous studies, suggesting that, even though most developed countries have made strides in reducing tobacco consumption, cigarette smoking remains one of the world's major killers.

Today, tobacco marketers spend $18 for every dollar spent on tobacco-control programs.[14] Maintaining anti-smoking gains to date, and making further inroads, may well become more difficult as every additional smoker becomes that much more valuable to hard-pressed cigarette makers. We don't have to look to the future, though, to appreciate the imperative of behavior modification today. If current smoking patterns continue, an estimated 5.6 million young people now alive will die prematurely.[15]

Physical Inactivity

Physical exercise protects against disease and can help to treat many chronic conditions.[16] One systematic literature review suggests that, each year, as many as five million deaths worldwide might be attributable to physical inactivity. In 2015 about 7 percent of early deaths from coronary disease, 7 percent of deaths from diabetes, and 10 percent of deaths from breast and colon cancer resulted from physical inactivity.[17] These are conservative estimates; the statistical models underlying them omit inactivity-linked risk factors such as obesity, high cholesterol, and high blood sugar.[18] On the whole, the World Health Organization estimates that physical inactivity is the fourth-leading cause of death globally.

On the other hand, ample evidence demonstrates that even a small amount of physical exercise is beneficial. A United Kingdom study of health-survey data collected between 1994 and 2016 grouped 63,591 participants into three categories: insufficiently active people, who engage in vigorous activity fewer than 75 minutes per week or moderate activity fewer than 150 minutes each week; weekend warriors, who exercise intensely one or twice a week for more than 150 minutes; and inactive people, who do no regular physical exercise. Compared with inactive participants, insufficiently active participants were 34 percent less likely to die from any cause and weekend warriors were 30 percent less likely. Even though insufficiently active adults and weekend warriors do not meet exercise guidelines, they enjoy significant health benefits.[19]

As we have seen, the life-expectancy effects of many traditional medical interventions are quite modest. In comparison, the effects of physical activity are potent. Evidence from the Cooper Institute for Exercise Studies in Dallas finds that regular joggers live, on average, three years longer than non-runners—even if the runners occasionally smoke cigarettes, consume alcohol, or are overweight. Aggregating data from existing studies, the researchers discovered that regular running, regardless of pace, reduces risk of premature mortality by 40 percent. One way to think of it is that an hour of running yields up to seven hours in increased life expectancy. Other forms of exercise such as walking and cycling also reduce the risk of premature death, but not to the same extent as running.[20]

A variety of studies also show that cognitive decline associated with aging can be slowed or even reversed by physical activity.

One meta-analysis of thirty studies in which otherwise-inactive individuals were assigned to exercise programs found that only 22 percent of those not assigned to exercise programs were able to maintain the level of cognitive functioning of the average person assigned to exercise.[21]

Poor Diet

On average, Americans consume about five pounds of food per day. That is seventy-three tons in the course of an eighty-year lifetime. Our choices about what goes into all those tons can have significant impact on our health and well-being.

In many developing countries—and in the United States until the 1940s—most diet-related diseases result from malnutrition and under-consumption of calories.[22] These diseases include rickets, caused by vitamin D deficiency; pellagra, from lack of niacin (a B vitamin); scurvy, from inadequate vitamin C; beri-beri, a result of deficient thiamine (also a B vitamin); and goiter, caused by iodine shortage. Public-health efforts have largely eliminated many of these diseases. For instance, after it became apparent that goiters were associated with a lack of iodine, salt iodization largely solved the problem in developed countries.

Lately the concern has been not so much scarcity as super-abundance, resulting in serious weight problems. According to the Centers for Disease Control and Prevention, the prevalence of obesity in the United States increased 74 percent between 1991 and 2001. In 2010 at least a quarter of the people in thirty-six states were obese. In a dozen other states, more than 30 percent of the people were obese.[23] Obesity is a problem affecting young and old: about 17 percent of Americans between the ages of 2 and 19 are obese, and it has been estimated that more than 300,000 US adults die of obesity-related causes each year.[24] Obesity also reduces quality of life. Sufferers face functional limitations such as travel restrictions and inability to walk as far and fast as others in their age group. Some need assistance with activities of daily living. In 2002, weight-related problems were responsible for more than 9 percent of US health care expenditures, more than $92 billion.[25] Some estimate that the annual individual cost of medical care for the obese is about $1,900 more than for individuals of normal weight.[26]

One need not be obese to be dangerously overweight. Using body mass index as a metric, 69 percent of American adults are considered to be at least overweight. Blacks and Latinos are at greater risk than whites.[27] About a third of Americans aged between 2 and 19 are overweight.[28] They are likely to continue having weight problems as adults—problems that contribute to the development of coronary disease, stroke, and high blood pressure, as well as diabetes, cancers, and arthritis.[29]

Medical interventions such as bariatric surgery can help overweight and obese people achieve healthy weight. But, on the whole, biomedicine does not have much to offer overweight people, except therapies to try to deal with the diseases, injuries, and other complications resulting from weight problems. The best choices for such people—the sorts of choices that do the most to improve health and quality of life—are not therapies but behavioral changes. In particular, exercising, if possible, and eating healthfully.

The latter is not at all simple, though, owing to the psychological challenges of eating well, the deficiencies that poverty can impose on diets, and the scarcity of nutrition in so-called food deserts (neighborhoods underserved by high-quality grocers). The availability of good food is a complex problem. Grocers will provide what sells. High-quality food is also higher in cost, placing it out of range for many customers. Of course, some people would prefer to buy lettuce but settle on nearby liquor instead. And, while certain rules of thumb are helpful, just what constitutes a good diet is often disputed. The best of intentions can be foiled by bad advice, of which there is a great deal when it comes to nutrition. Many popular diets have never been rigorously tested.

The Mediterranean diet is an exception: a behavioral intervention known, through solid research, to have positive health effects. The program replicates the consumption patterns of traditional cultures in Crete, Greece, and southern Italy. Those partaking of the Mediterranean diet obtain less than 8 percent of their calories from saturated fat, with all fats accounting for between 25 and 35 percent of calories. This diet is rich in fruits, vegetables, whole grains, olive oil, beans, nuts, legumes, seeds, herbs, and spices. Fish, including shellfish, is the principal source of animal protein, followed by smaller helpings of poultry, eggs, cheese, and yogurt. Water is the preferred beverage, along with wine in moderation.[30]

Each component of the Mediterranean diet has been researched extensively, to determine effects on risk factors for cardiovascular disease. Consumption of olive oil, as compared to animal fats, is related to lower LDL cholesterol and higher HDL cholesterol. Evidence suggests that adherence to a Mediterranean diet can reduce the risk of metabolic syndrome, lower the risk of diabetes and insulin resistance, and improve endothelial function. The diet also can reduce oxidative stress, which can hinder natural cell-repair mechanisms. The Mediterranean diet is also believed to reduce the risk of hypertension and arterial stiffness.[31] A study involving 15,152 participants from 52 countries found that daily consumption of fruits and vegetables, key components of the Mediterranean diet, was associated with a 30 percent reduction in the risk of a heart attack.[32] A study involving 93,122 US women found that following the Mediterranean diet was associated with a 36 percent reduction in the risk of sudden cardiac death.[33]

The Mediterranean diet also has been linked to better overall health outcomes. One meta-analysis with an aggregated sample size of 1,574,299 suggests that consumption of the Mediterranean diet is associated with at least a 9 percent reduction in premature mortality from any cause.[34] Another study, of 22,043 people living in Greece, finds that adherence to the Mediterranean diet is associated with a 25 percent reduction in premature all-cause mortality.[35] A more recent study built statistical models based on the National Health and Nutrition Examination Survey and a systematic analysis of major clinical trials and observational studies. Researchers found that an abnormally high or low intake of just ten foods or nutrients was associated with 45 percent of the premature deaths from heart disease, stroke, and diabetes in the United States. The study suggested the intake of fruits, vegetables, nuts and seeds, whole grains, polyunsaturated fats, and seafood omega-3 fats should be increased and that unprocessed red meats, processed meats, sugar-sweetened beverages, and sodium should be decreased.[36]

Disparities in dietary quality persist, despite well-intentioned efforts to ameliorate them. For example, the Supplemental Nutrition Assistance Program (SNAP) is the largest food assistance in the United States. One study evaluated the quality of diets among 38,969 adults, including 6,162 SNAP participants, 6,692 adults with incomes comparable to SNAP participants but who did not participate in SNAP, and 25,842 adults with high incomes. All groups were evaluated in eight cycles of the National Health and Nutrition Examination Survey between 1999 and 2017. Overall diets became healthier during this interval. But SNAP participants were significantly less likely to improve their diets in comparison to income matched non-participants and higher-income individuals. SNAP participants consumed more processed food, refined sugars, and fewer nuts and seeds.[37]

Behavior: The Bottom Line

Drug abuse, smoking, lack of exercise, and poor diet are just some of the behaviors that lead to poor health. Data from a committee of the Society of Behavioral Medicine offers a brief overview of what we know about strong links between behavior and health (see Appendix, Behavior-Health Linkages among Major "Actual Causes" of Death and Major Diseases). Many of these findings show that, even among people genetically predisposed to health problems, behavior is a crucial precursor to health outcomes.[38] The long, tedious appendix is included to make a point: the amount of evidence supporting behavioral interventions is very substantial.

Can Behavior Be Changed?

Although there is plenty of evidence that behavior affects health outcomes, the question remains, can anything be done about it? When it comes to physical exercise, there are competing priorities to worry about: family, career, hobbies. Time for self-improvement is limited. As for diet and smoking, the psychological challenges of reform are substantial. Bad habits are hard to break, and good ones equally difficult to cultivate. A healthful diet may also be financially inaccessible to poor people, a social problem as much as a behavioral one.

Given these obstacles, it is reasonable to question whether we can really expect more from behavioral change than we have gotten from biomedicine alone. While no one would doubt that individuals can do better, skepticism toward the possibility of beneficial large-scale shifts is understandable. And yet the evidence is all around us. One shining example is the prohibition of smoking in public places. These bans demonstrate unequivocally the capacity of policy to modify behavior in ways that improve health at the level of nations. A meta-analysis of studies published between January 2004 and April 2009 finds that, overall, US communities that passed smoking bans experienced a 17 percent reduction in acute heart attacks. Although these bans don't necessarily cause people to quit, they greatly reduce exposure to secondhand smoke, which can increase the risk of an acute heart attack by 30 percent.[39]

Public policy and citizen action can also change people's dietary patterns for the better. For instance, evidence shows that public health interventions can reduce consumption of trans fats.[40] These fats—common in baked goods, crackers, margarines, and deep-fried foods—can significantly increase the risk of death from heart disease.[41] As awareness of the dangers of trans fats has grown, populations have demanded responses from government and industry, leading not only to legal changes but also to healthier products.[42]

The power of public policy has been demonstrated all over the world. Turkey cut down on smoking rates after enacting an anti-tobacco law in 1996, which was followed by additional legislation in 2004 and 2008. The laws enlarged the size of health-warning labels on cigarette packages, dramatically increased cigarette taxes, and banned tobacco advertising, including event sponsorship. Between 2008 and 2012, smoking declined in Turkey by 13.4 percent.[43] In the year after Hungary imposed a tax on sugar, salt, and caffeine, 40 percent of manufacturers there changed product formulas to reduce use of the taxed ingredients. As a result, at least one in four Hungarians reduced their consumption of these products by 25–35 percent.[44]

And the one-peso-per-liter tax Mexico placed on sugar-sweetened beverages on New Year's Day, 2014, led to a 7.6 percent reduction in consumption of such drinks by the end of 2015. The largest decline was observed among lower-income groups at greatest risk for obesity and tooth decay.[45] The World Health Organization has been a major force in urging these sorts of policies and is working on similar projects in more than 150 countries.[46]

Along with impressive observational data, high-quality clinical research data show the benefits of behavioral change. Skeptics have downplayed the rigor of behavioral research; for instance, Marcia Angell and Arnold Relman, the former editors of the *New England Journal of Medicine*, claimed that "the literature contains very few scientifically sound studies of the relation, if there is one, between mental state and disease."[47] But, as my colleague Veronica Irvin and I have shown, such studies are at least as reliable as their pharmacological counterparts.[48] We reviewed every large clinical trial carried out between 1980 and 2012 supported by either the National Heart, Lung, and Blood Institute (NHLBI) or the National Institute of Diabetes and Digestive and Kidney Diseases.[49] Reports from behavioral trials met a high methodological standard: three-fourths of trials were registered at ClinicalTrials.gov, a new federal service that requires investigators to declare their hypotheses and outcome measures before collecting data. This promotes rigorous research standards. Eighty-four percent of registered behavioral trials reported an objectively measured physiological outcome. Among these, 81 percent reported a significant benefit from behavioral intervention. In randomized trials, the gold standard in medical research, behavioral interventions were associated with prevention of diabetes, improved blood-pressure control, weight loss, and reduced hospital readmission.

These benefits are heartening, but they tell only part of the story about the effects of behavioral change. As with biomedical interventions, behavioral interventions should be able to demonstrate improvements not only in surrogate markers but also in longevity and quality of life. It isn't enough to know that people are smoking less, eating more healthfully, or getting more regular exercise. We need to know that they are living longer, healthier lives.

Irvin and I found that behavioral trials have some way to go when it comes to addressing morbidity and mortality. About 45 percent of the trials we documented reported morbidity outcomes. Among these, 18 percent reported a significant benefit. About 24 percent of behavioral trials assessed mortality, and all were null for this outcome.[50] While these numbers don't look very inspiring, we should keep in mind that traditional medical trials rarely show significant benefit for morbidity and mortality outcomes. The morbidity benefits observed in behavioral trials were in line with those observed in trials of pharmaceutical interventions.[51] And, as discussed in Chapter 3, our NHLBI review identified no trials—behavioral or biomedical—published between 2000 and 2014 that documented a significant reduction in all-cause mortality.

This is not, of course, an invitation to behavioral researchers to rest on their laurels. The deficits of some biomedical research should not be the standard for any behavioral research. Scientists, policy-makers, and the public should demand high-quality clinical science from researchers working in every area of health care. And what we do know about behavioral intervention should convince us that it is worth such rigorous investigation.

Unfortunately, NIH does not appear to agree. In the late 1980s and early 1990s, both House and Senate appropriators put pressure on the NIH to bring the level of funding for behavioral and social science research to above 10 percent of the NIH budget. Sandra Scarr, testifying in 1989 before Congress as the president of the American Psychological Association, estimated that the NIH spent only about 3.17 percent of its budget on behavioral and social science research.[52] Over the next few years, members of House and Senate appropriations committees repeatedly raised concerns about the low level of support for behavioral research, suggesting that 10 percent of the NIH budget would be appropriate.[53] NIH director Bernadine Healy told a congressional hearing that she agreed with the 10 percent target.[54] In response to questioning from the appropriators, Dr. Healy required all NIH institutes to develop a ten-year plan for behavioral research. But, she challenged the low estimate of NIH funding for behavioral research, arguing that the real problems was a poor accounting system. It has now been thirty years since the NIH promised Congress that they would increase the proportion of NIH funds devoted to social and behavioral sciences. How well has this strategy worked?

It is not easy to track these expenditures. Over two decades after NIH promised better accounting of their research expenditures, they rolled out the Research, Condition, and Disease Categorization (RCDC) system, which assigns each NIH grant to one or more of 264 possible categories. RCDC reports that funding for the behavioral and social sciences research category is not near the bottom of the distribution of funding across the 264 categories, with an expenditure of $3.6 billion in 2015. According to the public access website, it appears spending on behavioral and social sciences research is similar to investments in brain disorders or on pediatrics. So, why all the fuss?

The problem is in the details of the methodology. Using RCDC, computer programs read the grants to identify how often the keywords are used. If the frequency of the words used is above a threshold value, 100 percent of the dollars for that grant is placed in that category. The problem is that grants can be placed into more than one category. If a grant is placed into five different categories, the same budget is counted five different times. The bizarre accounting scheme, which double-, triple-, even quintuple-counts grant values, allows the $25 billion research budget to report it is funding $160 billion in grants.

NIH knew about this problem and commissioned an internal study to estimate actual expenditures.[55] A copy of the study was obtained through a Freedom of Information Act request. A new methodology was developed to estimate the proportion of the total effort in each grant that was true behavioral and social sciences research. For example, consider a grant on the management of type 2 diabetes. The grant might have a small component on behavioral intervention for weight loss. The RCDC method is likely to attribute 100 percent of the budget for the grant to the behavioral category. In addition, it would have attributed 100 percent of the budget to the diabetes category, 100 percent of the budget to the obesity category and 100 percent of the budget to the nutrition category. Instead of counting the entire grant in multiple categories, the new method estimated the percentage of the total effort for each of the subcategories, using a method wherein the different components could not add up to more than 100 percent.

The study used data from fiscal year 2011, when the official RCDC system suggested that behavioral and social sciences research accounted for $3.4 billion. Dividing this by the NIH actual research budget gave an estimate that behavioral research accounted for about 15 percent of the NIH budget. However, this is clearly a gross overestimate of actual expenditures for behavioral and social science research. The new method suggests that the correct investment is about $600 million, or about 2.4 percent of the NIH research budget.[56] Assuming that behavior and social circumstances account for about half the variance in health outcome, this seems like a very small expenditure.

As the study demonstrated, behavioral, social, and public health research constitute a very small part of its research portfolio. One analysis suggested that in fiscal year 2014, grants including the terms "gene," "genome," or "genetic" received about 50 percent more support than those that make no mention of genes but use the term "prevention." Between 2004 and 2014, the proportion of NIH-funded projects including the terms "public" or "population" in their titles declined by about 90 percent.[57]

What about Physician Behavior?

So far, I have focused on what individuals, public institutions, and scientists can do to improve health outcomes through behavioral change. Health providers have a large role to play, too. Unfortunately, they are leaving a lot of potential benefits on the table.

With my colleague Glenn Morgan from the National Cancer Institute, I recently examined data from the nationally representative Medical Expenditures Panel Survey (MEPS), which asks participants about preventive services they have received. Even though smoking is clearly the most important factor in premature death, in the year preceding the interview, only about half of adult smokers reported having been advised by a physician to quit. Men 18 to 44 years old with less education and relatively low incomes are especially likely to be smokers, yet this group was rarely advised to quit. More than 65 percent of male smokers older than 65 were advised to quit, compared with 31 percent of younger men (ages 18–44). Hispanic respondents were also less likely to be advised to quit (33 percent) than were white non-Hispanics (49 percent), even though the former experience a disproportionate share of poor outcomes associated with cigarette use. Doctors in the Northeast, where smoking is less common, advised 56 percent of patients to quit, whereas doctors in the South, where smoking rates are relatively high, gave the same advice to just 44 percent of patients.[58] When physicians did advise patients to stop smoking, they usually did not recommend evidence-based interventions, which have been shown in various studies to boost the number of successful quit attempts by anywhere from 24 to 60 percent.[59] Perhaps this is why, in the study, smokers advised to quit did not have better quit rates than those who were not so advised.

Doctors may be grudging when it comes to smoking-cessation advice, but they are effusive about medical screening. Nearly all of the survey respondents reported that doctors had in the previous year advised them to receive screening for cancers and other diseases. This despite the modest effects of screening on health outcomes—far more modest than the benefits of smoking cessation, as noted previously.

Doctors also could do more to promote regular physical activity. MEPS data on exercise advice are a mixed bag. On the one hand, between 2002 and 2010, black Americans increasingly reported receiving counsel to exercise more; on the other hand, no improvement was reported in the rate advice was given to white or Hispanic respondents. Overall, in each year of the survey, no more than 60 percent of respondents reported that a physician had advised them to exercise more. In a country where seven in ten residents are overweight, doctors should not be so hesitant to urge patients toward better physical fitness.

Conclusion

It should be obvious that behavior is a key determinant of health. Human genetics haven't changed much in the past million or so years, but our survivability has. That is because we have learned to do things differently. To use medical science, yes, but also to treat ourselves better through improved sanitation and food safety, reduced food scarcity, better working conditions, and the dissemination of healthful practices.

Indeed, to most of us all this *is* obvious. And yet the nexus of government, academic, and corporate institutions responsible for studying health and health interventions, and delivering those interventions, treats this common sense as an afterthought. Perhaps that is in the nature of common sense: no one owns it, which means no one can gain credit for it. But scientists can do, and have done, good studies of it. Taking their research seriously is an important step toward a balanced health care system centered on patients rather than treatments.

7

A Way Forward

If pressed to name science's defining, guiding principle, one could do worse than "respect for the evidence." Without empirical findings—the more the better—we can make no claims. And what claims we make must also be plausible, in light of the evidence. Among other things, this means we strive to adjust our beliefs as the evidence demands. When evidence changes, so should our views.

For more than seven decades, the prevailing view among Americans has been that health is achieved overwhelmingly through medical intervention to prevent and heal sickness. The biomechanism is understood as inherently functioning, but also subject to wear, breakage, and sabotage by pathogens. Fortunately, through clinical application of the fruits of biomedical science, the biomechanism could be restored or hardened.

This was a reasonable paradigm for the pursuit of health at the end of World War II. Communicable disease was on the decline in wealthy countries, and chronic disease had not yet entered the public consciousness as a great scourge. This good fortune seemed self-evidently a result of scientific and technological advances such as the discovery and mass production of antibiotics and vaccines and the development of improved surgical techniques.

Today, however, we should be prepared to reexamine the biomedical paradigm. Medicine and medical science are undoubtedly useful, but a growing body of evidence suggests that, in the United States, we have reached a point of diminishing returns with respect to population health. We will continue to figure out clever ways to treat individual diseases. But if we want to improve lives and save money at a national scale, we need to do more than treat disease. We need to foster health.

Too many Americans believe we are already up to that task. I don't assert that they are wrong, but let us at least test their faith. Consider the evidence against. Peer countries that devote more resources to social services and less to health care consistently experience better longevity results, and the performance gap is widening. US death rates are increasing, especially in the most deprived segments of society.[1] Medicine has done very little to reduce the dramatic inequities in health outcomes.[2] Our biomedical moonshots routinely disappoint,[3] even as other investments, much more likely to foster health, are starved of funding.[4] Most important, high expectations for medical intervention have been used to justify almost unlimited expenditures on medical technologies, allowing US medical care to consume nearly one in every five dollars spent on goods and services.[5] These high expenditures have consequences. Because so much is spent on health care, less is available to spend on the defense, roads, education, transportation, and other vital services.[6] Health care confiscates resources that are needed to achieve the American dream.

Few of these claims are controversial among scholars in public health and medicine.[7] They are based in evidence, most of it produced in the past three or so decades. Life scientists, physicians, social scientists, and statisticians have questioned the wisdom of our narrow investment in biomedical approaches to health.[8] The results of their inquiries counsel change—new attitudes, policies, and scientific priorities.[9] But change is slow in coming.

It is not my contention that biomedicine is inherently harmful or useless. Far from it. It is my contention that researchers and the wider citizenry should continually debate strategies for extracting public benefit from scientific knowledge. I believe that an open debate, accountable to the latest evidence, will inspire significant reforms.

A Vision for the Future

If the narrative about biomedical research and health care is not completely reliable, how might we revise priorities to improve population health? In the Introduction, I reviewed Eugene Steuerle's assertion that many of our funding priorities were set by men (and a few women) who have been dead for decades.[10] Once patterns of spending are implemented, they achieve a life of their own. For most agencies, this year's budget looks pretty much like last year's budget, with a few minor adjustments. And, health spending is an oversized component of the US economy. To make the population healthier, we need a new vision of health, biomedical research, and health care. A big order indeed.

What might a reenvisioned health research and health care system look like? In the remainder of this chapter, I consider the evidence that relatively modest investments might have big effects on the life expectancies and quality of life of American citizens. I explore how changing the way we fund health care and biomedical research might save a substantial number of lives, reduce harm associated with health care, and significantly reduce the cost of care.

The Definition of Health: From
Biomarkers to Patient Centeredness

Why are there such different interpretations of the same studies on the effects of medical treatments? Women may feel that getting regular mammograms protects them against death from breast cancer, or people may understand that taking a statin drug will prevent death from heart disease.[11] Critics argue that the value of these preventive actions is very modest.[12] Women who get regular mammograms do die of breast cancer, and there are plenty of deaths from heart disease among people who take cholesterol-lowering medications.[13] The preventive actions may change the probability of these outcomes, but only slightly.

The difference in outlook can be explained by our focus of attention. The goal of medical care is not exclusively to have people use more health services.[14] These services are tools to help us achieve one of two patient-centered goals: longer life, and better life quality during the years we live. These goals should always be at the forefront of our interest.

Take the statin trials that evaluate the most commonly prescribed medications in the United States. Worldwide, lipid-regulating drug sales hit a peak of $39.1 billion in 2011. Since then, several of the leading products have gone off patent, but sales remain above $25 billion per year. Systematic randomized clinical trials very consistently demonstrate that statin medications lower cholesterol, and there is tremendous enthusiasm for near-universal use of these medicines.[15] But cholesterol is a surrogate marker; it stands in for the risk of early death. In the best clinical trials of these medications, the chances of living longer, as measured by all-cause mortality, are often unaffected. For example, the large ASPEN clinical trial showed that 4.6 percent of those taking a statin died within the four-year study follow-up assessment, compared with 4.3 percent of those randomly assigned to the comparison group.[16] In the AFCAPS/TexCAPS clinical trial, 2.4 percent of those randomly assigned to take statins died during the five-year study period, in contrast to 2.3 percent in the comparison group.[17]

There are different ways of looking at the risks and benefits of medical care. Focusing on different goals allows different interpretations of the value of treatment. I prefer to keep attention focused on the bottom line: the quality and quantity of life of the people health care serves. From evaluating medical care to setting the criteria for licensing new medications, we need to keep focus on the bottom line. Attention needs to remain on benefits and harms, from the patient's perspective.

Research: From Mechanism to Outcome

Are our expenditures on biomedical research the most efficient way to identify maneuvers that will help people live longer healthier lives? More precisely, do we have the best allocation of resources across basic, clinical, and public-health research to achieve the goals of better population health?

Should we give up any aspect of research, basic, clinical, or public health? Certainly not! Basic science funding remains crucial. Continued advances in genetics, immunology, and control of infectious disease need public and private support. New advances in genetics-based noninvasive diagnoses are revolutionizing prenatal risk detection using DNA captured from maternal blood.[18] These advances have played a central role in improving the human condition. But the most recent evidence also underscores the value of clinical, social, behavioral, and public-health sciences; each makes important contributions to knowledge and to the development of future treatment. But is our formula for allocating these resources correct? Our current model puts nearly all the eggs in the basic-science basket, and may tell us more about the power of vested interest groups than about the likelihood that various lines of research are in the best interest of those who pay for it. Basic biomedical science needs to coexist with other scholarship that informs our understanding of life expectancy and quality of life. Just as developments in basic life sciences are too important to ignore, so are developments in the social and public-health sciences documenting the profound impact of social factors on human health.[19] Investments should be coordinated with the long-term goal of improving population health.[20]

We need more attention paid to lines of research that do not fit the traditional narrative: enough evidence has accumulated to justify support for a broader range of research. It is true that the current portfolio includes both basic and social science. Yet, as noted in Chapter 6, the behavioral and social science investment may be less that 3 percent of the total expenditure, while the effects of behavioral and social factors may explain half the variation in health outcomes. To improve human health, it may be necessary to change the allocation, with more effort devoted to learning how social and clinical science can be applied to prevention and clinical care. As a start, the investment should be increased to at least the intended 10 percent level.

Philosophy of Science: Treat the
Narrative as Scientific Theory

The NIH vision statement is "Turning Discovery into Cure." That is how we sell biomedical research. Textbooks explain that there is a known way to eradicate disease. It begins with identifying biological pathogens, followed by the systematic creation of a medicine to destroy the pathogen and eliminate the threat. Or a metabolic error is identified and corrected. When a person stops making insulin, the missing hormone can be replaced with injections. Although this strategy saves lives for conditions such as insulin-dependent diabetes, it works for only a limited number of health problems.

Science progresses most when citizens and scientists continually evaluate and reevaluate ideas. The narrative about the current trajectory of biomedical research, the benefits of medical care, and the importance of social determinants of health will continue to be debated. Fostering different perspectives and motivated advocates is healthy. When evaluating differences of opinion, we should keep focused on the data and methods used to support the conclusions.

As the discussion advances, it will be important to keep the fighting fair. There's no shortage of physicians and scientists unimpressed with claims for the value of popular therapies.[21] The narrative is like any other scientific theory: objective tests of its value can be constructed and executed. This book has argued that many aspects of the narrative are not clearly supported by the data. Others may disagree, and advocates for the different positions may use different data and different tests. That is how science works. We should be prepared to use the best objective evidence to fuel the discussion and to keep the discussion transparent. I hope I have convinced you that there are plenty of reasons to doubt the predominant narrative about the pathway from basic science laboratories to near-term clinical cures.

Scientific Reporting: From Selective
Reporting to Transparent Disclosure

Many of the problems highlighted in this book are the result of inadequate or hidden research information. Much of what we have learned about the limitations of the narrative has resulted from greater transparency requirements. Until relatively recently, research investigators measured numerous outcome variables but reported only those that were statistically significant. In many cases, if the results did not support their ideas, the investigators did not report anything at all. Or, when evaluations of new treatments were negative, we were not granted access to the results. When scientific standards changed to require greater transparency in the registration and reporting of research studies, we began to learn that many promising medical interventions were not that promising after all.[22]

Transparency is an important tool for revealing the truth. Recently, the NIH initiated a new policy that would require prospective registration of human studies. Registration assumes that hypotheses are laid out in advance and that investigators declare their primary outcome variables; this limits the reporting of outcomes that are likely attributable to chance. Further, registration helps identify studies that did not find a significant treatment effect. It saves resources by assuring that the same studies are not done over and over again. Even though truthful transparent reporting sounds like a no-brainer, the scientific community has not eagerly jumped on board. In response to the new policy on transparency, more than 3,500 scientists signed a letter in opposition.[23]

Greater transparency in the regulation of pharmaceutical and medical products is also necessary. For example, the US Food and Drug Administration (FDA) is the most important regulator of drugs and devices in the United States. The FDA also sets the standard for other parts of the world. Until relatively recently, the detailed and complex decision processes used by the FDA were not easily accessible by the public. Other regulators, including the European Medicines Agency, have adopted policies that make the enormous amount of information used to make regulation decisions available to the public. This is necessary because some of the most crucial information is hidden from public view. For example, the FDA sees data from clinical trials when a manufacturer attempts to get a product license. One analysis identified seven cases in which a pharmaceutical product caused higher death rates than the comparison medication or placebo. These higher death rates were disclosed to the public in only one case.[24] A recent book by medical journalist Jeanne Lenzer describes efforts to determine the safety of implanted medical devices. She describes numerous cases of harmful reactions to approved devices. In many of the cases, harmful and in some cases fatal reactions were not clearly disclosed to the public or to physicians using the devices.[25]

To address this issue, research investigators from a variety of different institutions created the "Blueprint for Transparency at FDA." The group made eighteen recommendations based on five principles. The principles included disclosing more information about milestones in the application process, disclosing more about how the FDA makes decisions, disclosing more information about the application and review process, correcting misleading information, and offering greater disclosure about the scientific studies that led to the product licenses.[26]

Transparency is a cornerstone of good science. In particular, citizens depend on the FDA to protect them, and it is important that principles of disclosure be applied. The new 21st Century Cures Act does little to encourage transparency. In fact, it leaves in place several of the provisions that allow data to be hidden from the public, while emphasizing the need to get drugs to market quickly.

Purpose of Health Care: From Find and Fix to Prevent, Promote, and Care

Neal Halfon, my former collaborator at UCLA, and colleagues described three systems of health care (Table 7.1).[27] The first, System 1.0, emerged in the nineteenth century, maturing while germ theory was the dominant scientific explanation for the sources of illness. Health care focused on acute infectious diseases and was delivered in hospitals—"doctors workshops,"[28] where broken people would be diagnosed and, hopefully, repaired.

Table 7.1 Neal Halfon's three systems of health care

Characteristics of system	Health System 1.0 (Yesterday)	Health System 2.0 (Today)	Health System 3.0 (Tomorrow)
Focus	Acute and infectious disease	Chronic disease	Optimal health
Foundational theory	Germ theory	Multiple risk factors	Complex systems—life course pathways
Time frame considered	Short	Longer	Lifespan / generational
Services offered	Medical care	Chronic disease management and prevention	Heterogeneous services coordinated across sectors
Financing model	Insurance-based financing	Prepaid benefits	Investment in population-based prevention
Delivery model	Industrial	Corporate	Network
Goal	Reducing deaths	Prolonging disability-free life	Producing optimal health for all

Source: Courtesy of Neal Halfon, UCLA Center for Children, Families, and Communities.

This system worked well enough that by the middle of the twentieth century, the problem of acute, communicable disease had receded. System 2.0, the postwar model, focused on non-communicable, chronic illness. The source of health care delivery shifted from hospitals to primary care clinics, where biological diagnostics designed in professional laboratories were used to identify and manage long-term risk factors.[29]

But while the differences between System 1.0 and 2.0 were vast, an essential similarity linked them: both were based on the assumption that pathogens are responsible for most diseases. Since the late twentieth century, however, research has made an older truth impossible for scientists to ignore: health outcomes are products of complicated ecologies implicating socioeconomic and behavioral conditions, no less than biological ones.[30]

It is therefore time, Halfon argues, for something new—System 3.0. This will not be a health care system but instead a health system. In this system of the future, the emphasis shifts from treatment of illness and risk factors to achieving optimal health. Pathogens and risk factors are not alien to System 3.0, but neither is the rest of life. Rather than confine itself to the sick, the system promotes health across the lifespan.[31] The goal is not just to have a cure for every disease, but to foster the wellness of every person. We will test success by the health of our population, not by approval of the latest prohibitively expensive drug.

This shift involves a change of mind-set. We will still look to health care as a means of promoting wellness, but we will also look to schools, social services, and environmental regulatory agencies. Ensuring our children's health will no longer mean just getting them immunizations and checkups, but also reading to them, applying appropriate discipline, and enrolling them in pre-school programs. These interventions are known to improve the trajectory of whole lives.[32] They can also be expensive, but, compared with chronic care, prevention is cheap.[33]

Indeed, a study in the *New England Journal of Medicine* by Jarett Berry and colleagues shows how important it is to account for the whole life course. The researchers aggregated evidence from eighteen cohort studies involving 257,384 adult participants and focused on 72,811 men and women who were 55 or younger when they entered the studies. Investigators found that people who had not developed any heart disease risk factors by age 55 had a substantially lower risk of dying of heart disease by age 80. Fifty-five-year-old male nonsmokers who had avoided high blood pressure, high cholesterol, and diabetes had a 3.6 percent lifetime risk of heart attack; men with two or more major risk factors had a 37.5 percent chance of experiencing heart attack. Fifty-five-year-old women with no risk factors had a 1 percent risk of experiencing heart attacks, compared with 18.3 percent of women with two or more of the major risk factors.[34]

Other studies have shown that people who were overweight or obese early in life continued to gain weight throughout life. When compared forty years later with peers who had not been overweight as children, those with early weight problems had significantly worse physical functioning.[35]

The benefits of a healthful life trajectory extend beyond avoiding death from chronic killers, including the ability to participate in activities of daily living throughout the lifespan, as well as delaying the onset of symptoms and disabilities. These benefits reduce both the time spent suffering and the cost of extending life. For instance, one analysis suggested Alzheimer's patients who can delay long-term care by five years may save as much as a half million dollars each.[36]

A health care system attempts to restore us when our bodies break. A health system is a lifelong process of cultivating wellness, so that the body is less prone to breaking early. Realizing the latter will demand the effort of scientists and citizens.

Range of Tools: From Clinic to Public Policy

Under System 3.0, we will think more creatively about how to use law to improve health by helping ensure access to decent housing and education.

One area in which we can do better is the prevention and remediation of homelessness. Estimating how many homeless people are in the United States is difficult, but the best evidence puts the number around 550,000. Among these, about a third live without shelter, meaning that they lack even temporary housing provided by charitable and social services. About 35 percent of the homeless are families with children.[37] Homelessness is associated with a wide range of health problems, often exacerbated by chronic mental illness.[38] Evidence suggests that the life expectancy of homeless people is about fifty years, roughly thirty fewer than that of non-homeless Americans. Homeless people 45–64 years old are 4.5 times more likely to die from any cause than are members of the general population.[39]

A legislator in Hawaiʻi—which, according to the National Alliance to End Homelessness, has the country's highest rate of homelessness—recently put forward an innovative proposal for tackling homelessness as a precursor of poor health. State senator Josh Green, an emergency room physician, has proposed allowing doctors to identify homelessness as a medical condition. They could write prescriptions for housing. Early analysis suggests this approach would save on Medicaid bills.[40] For example, one analysis by Helping Hands, a Hawai'i nonprofit organization, estimated that, once housed, medical expenses for the homeless decline by 43 percent.[41] As of this writing, legislation is working its way through the state legislature. In March 2017 it was deferred for more information, but remained alive in the process. Others, writing in traditional medical journals, argue that spending on homeless shelters makes good sense from both a medical and a financial perspective.[42]

Other accumulating evidence shows that investments in social services reduce health care costs. One example concerns area agencies on aging (AAAs). These agencies, which operate in many US counties, provide social services for senior citizens. The aging agencies differ from one another in their formal relationships with health care. In some cases, formal collaborations have been established between the aging agencies and health care provider groups. In other communities, these relationships are less formal. Using data from a national survey of aging agencies, Amanda Brewster and her colleagues at Yale compared hospital readmissions in communities that had either formal or informal relationships between the AAAs and health care providers,[43] They found that hospital readmissions were significantly lower in communities that had formal ties between the health care system and the social service sector. In addition, nursing home placements were significantly lower in communities where the AAA had programs that help divert unnecessary nursing home stays.

These findings demonstrate how investments in social services save money for the health care system. The problem, of course, is that the money comes out of different pockets. Raising and spending money in AAAs saves money for the health care system. In a coordinated system, money should be directly diverted from the health care system to the social service system. Under these circumstances, everyone benefits: the health care system would have lower costs, the social service system would be able to function more efficiently, and patients would have better outcomes. Unfortunately, there are too few examples of transfer of assets between these different entities.[44]

Policy-makers usually want to avoid paying for something that could come from another agency's budget. That may be why health insurers, including Medicare and Medicaid, are reluctant to pay for nontraditional services. But, what if paying for these services actually benefited their bottom line? Sometimes relatively simple nonmedical intervention can significantly reduce medical care costs. One example is the Community Aging in Place, Advancing Better Living for Elders (CAPABLE) program for low-income older adults with functional limitations. These people are particularly expensive to care for in the medical care system. In part, the high cost occurs because the acute medical care system is not well equipped to deal with their needs. In the CAPABLE program, an interprofessional team that includes an occupational therapist, a nurse, and a handyman make home visits to identify strategies for overcoming functional limitations. Compared with a matched control group, participants in the CAPABLE program cost $867 per month less. The calculation includes the cost of the CAPABLE team.[45]

Better priorities at the agency level are also important. From 2009 until 2017, under the leadership of director Thomas Frieden, the Centers for Disease Control was a model in this respect. The CDC developed new initiatives and partnerships concentrated on six behavioral and health-quality issues linked with leading causes of illness, injury, disability, and death: smoking, teen pregnancy, HIV, surgical infections, injury prevention, and childhood obesity.

By the time Frieden left office, significant progress had been made in several areas. Whereas 20.5 percent of adults used tobacco in 2008, 15.1 percent did in 2015. There were 37.9 births per 1,000 female teens in 2009, compared with 22.3 per 1,000 in 2015. Diagnosis and awareness of HIV infections increased. The rate of central line–associated surgical site infections fell, although gains did not meet target levels. There were also some failures, primarily in reducing incidence of obesity among children and adolescents.[46] Given the lifelong hazards resulting from childhood obesity, we can only hope that CDC and its partners took useful lessons from that disappointing result, to be applied in future efforts.

From Discovery to Implementation

Transition from research findings into practice is always challenging. It is not enough to discover that a new approach has promise. Despite spending literally billions of dollars making minor modifications to effective drug treatments, we often pass up opportunities to get more health by simply getting better dissemination of treatments that we know provide benefit.

Our bookshelves are littered with well-tested strategies that might improve health while lowering costs. But the pathway from a promising new idea to its implementation is long and treacherous. The idea must be reviewed by peers, funded, investigated in systematic studies, integrated into research syntheses, and accepted through the development of evidence-based practice guidelines. On average this process takes seventeen years.[47] And the best examples of the successful seventeen-year dissemination process are for patented pharmaceutical products. The profit incentive lures companies into spending billions of dollars to ensure that doctors prescribe their products. There is no parallel for behavioral and social approaches. When there is little profit incentive, the seventeen-year time trajectory may be optimistic. A new field, known as implementation sciences, is only now beginning to tackle this problem.[48]

From Silos to Collaboration

As much as we encourage collaboration across fields of scientific inquiry, areas of scientific investigation remain widely separated in disciplinary silos. Scientific methods and languages are difficult to learn. We are housed in different buildings, read different journals, and attend different meetings. But new rays of hope are appearing. One example is the NIH All of Us initiative. This effort will enroll a minimum of one million volunteers, who are expected to be well or to have a wide range of diseases. Many of the diseases will be common, such as arthritis, diabetes, or heart disease. But with more than a million participants, there will also be enough people to study rare conditions. All of Us will gather information on a remarkable number of health determinants, ranging from environmental exposures to genetic factors and social factors. The study will develop measures of risk for a range of diseases based on environmental exposures, genetic factors, health behaviors, and complex interactions between individual risk factors and exposures to risks. The study will take advantage of data collection using mobile devices, such as cell phones. With assurance of participant privacy, data will be made available to a wide range of research investigators. Most importantly, the All of Us initiative will encourage new opportunities for cross-disciplinary research.[49]

Financing: How Can We Afford Doing More?

Throughout this book, I have argued that the United States would benefit from new research exploring the health effects of quality improvement, social conditions, and behavior. Existing evidence suggests that a health system designed on the basis of this research will improve health by attending to a broader range of health determinants. Happily, other wealthy countries already demonstrate that such a system is also less expensive than our own.[50] But even if reform saves money in the long run, it will cost a lot in the short term. Where will the funds come from? One possible source is money we could be saving by reducing waste in the health care system. In 2013, the Institute of Medicine estimated that inefficiencies cost us about $750 billion per year in that sector.[51] This suggests that roughly a quarter of health care expenditures yield no benefit.

Donald Berwick and Andrew Hackbarth have isolated six systemic pathologies responsible for this waste.[52] First, they point to failures in health care delivery. Unsafe care and lack of preventive services cost between $102 and $154 billion per year. Preventive services are far less expensive than later chronic care. And medical complications, many of which persist thanks to our failure to invest sufficiently in quality improvement, create further need of health care.

A second source of cost overruns is poor care coordination, another cause of complications and hospital readmissions. Improved coordination begins with better communication among health care providers. For a start, electronic medical records help, especially in preventing medication errors. These errors are less common in systems such as the Veterans Administration's health services, which use a standardized electronic-records format.[53] Care-coordination problems cost between $25 and $45 billion each year, according to Berwick and Hackbarth's estimate.

Third on Berwick and Hackbarth's list is the predilection for overtreatment, the total yearly cost of which they place between $158 and $226 billion. The care patients receive is often unnecessary and may be unsupported by evidence.[54] Patients are subjected to unneeded surgeries and a surfeit of antibiotics.[55] Dramatic inconsistencies in the quantity of care delivered across geographies suggest that provider discretion is running up costs.[56] For example, heroic end-of-life care is given more often in some regions than in others, even though demand for such care does not vary significantly across the United States.[57]

Fourth is administrative bloat. A substantial portion of health care cost results from the complexities of billing, inconsistent insurer policies, and convoluted formulas for identifying appropriate procedures and patients eligible for services. Provider groups need specialized personnel to deal with the range and complexity of payer practices, and the costs of these personnel are eventually taken up by patients themselves.

Clinicians argue that administrative costs are out of control. For instance, some have noted that the average doctor spends more than $40,000 per year collecting and reporting quality-improvement data. Overall, that is more than $15 billion each year.[58] It has been suggested that very little of the data provided through this expensive process are ever used.[59] As we have seen, quality improvement can be a lifesaving intervention. But some efforts have turned into runaway trains. We need to find ways to make quality-improvement research more efficient.

Berwick and Hackbarth estimate the total annual costs from administrative complexity at between $107 and $389 billion.

Other countries do not face such high costs, in large part because their health care delivery systems are more centralized.[60] Uniformity would simplify administration immensely, cutting costs.

Berwick and Hackbarth's fifth target is pricing, which accounts for between $84 and $178 billion in unnecessary spending each year. The cost of health care services in the United States is frequently irrational, bearing little relation to actual cost of delivery and seemingly unmoved by competitive pressures. The same service may be offered at any number of prices in assorted contexts, depending on contractual relationships between providers and payers. Those who are uninsured might be billed at a retail price ten times the price offered to third-party payers, even though providers do not expect to be paid this amount or need to be in order to cover costs.[61] In the United States, some medical tests cost an order of magnitude more than in other countries. Neither doctors nor patients are well informed about the costs of pharmaceuticals and their alternatives, leading to further unnecessary spending.[62]

Finally, the sixth source of waste is fraud and abuse, such as fake billing schemes, which attempt to game the system in order to reap profits for providers. Such cheating is rare, but the software and accounting services required for fraud and abuse prevention are enormously expensive. Berwick and Hackbarth estimate the total costs of fraud and compliance with prevention regulations at between $82 and $272 billion per year. Again, reducing administrative complexity and increasing centralization would create savings by reducing opportunities for fraud and the cost of preventing it.

In total, Berwick and Hackbarth place the cost of systemic failures between $558 and $1263 billion per year. These estimates (Figure 7.1) are based on data available in 2011, so it is likely that current numbers would be higher.

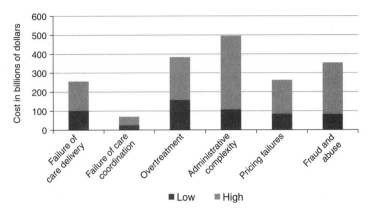

Figure 7.1. High and low estimates of costs of waste in health care, by category (in billions of 2011 US dollars), as calculated by Donald Berwick and Andrew Hackbarth. The bottom of each column represents the low estimate and the top the high estimate.

Eliminating all unnecessary and ineffective health services would yield a dividend approximately equal to the cost of US public education.[63] Such an outcome is too much to expect, but we can bite deeply into these wasteful expenditures without adversely affecting the health of the population. We could use some of the savings to fund scholarship that informs our understanding of the social and behavioral factors affecting individual and public health. The evidence we already have justifies supporting a broader range of research—more than can be furnished with only 3 percent of NIH grant money.

Plans Ready for Action

The strategies recommended by Berwick and Hackbarth remain fairly abstract. However, others have offered evidence-based plans that, if employed, might yield a significant level of savings.

Table 7.2 Strategies to reduce health care costs without risk to patients

Condition or problem	Cost per year	Strategy	Estimated cost savings per year
Late-stage cancer care	>$150 billion	Better formulation of goals Pain management Home or near-home chemotherapy	$37 billion
Chronic kidney disease management	$315 billion[a]	Aggressive early treatment Care coordination Alignment of care with patient preference, including home peritoneal dialysis	$63 billion
Stroke care	$48 billion	Rapid response teams to shorten time to deliver clot-dissolving medications Replacement of hospital care with high-quality home-based care Use of nurses to increase adherence to protective medications	$2.8 billion
Ambulatory surgical care	$209 billion	Use of decision aides targeted at overuse Expanded hours of surgical centers to 18 hours / day, 7 days / week Streamlined operations, better coordinated transitions	$45 billion
Spine care	$86 billion	Triage of low-risk patients Attention to both physical and psychosocial risks Use of shared decision-making tools	$21.5 billion
Critical care	$214 billion	Contactless monitors in non-ICU beds Mobile surveillance teams for rapid response Prevention of unnecessary ICU admissions (about 65% of all cases)	$42 billion
Obesity	$329 billion	Risk assessment and behavioral intervention Individually tailored weight-loss plans delivered by low-cost coaches Use of low-cost technologies to promote maintenance	$38 billion

a. 25% of Medicare budget

Source: Adapted from Stanford Medicine Clinical Excellence Research Center, http://med.stanford.edu/cerc/innovative-care-designs/care-delivery-designs.html.

The Clinical Excellence Research Center (CERC) at Stanford University has proposed a series of interventions that might lower cost without harm to patients. Each year, a group of fellows spends an academic year doing an in-depth exploration of a particular high-cost problem in health care delivery. The fellows, usually young physicians or PhD-level clinical scientists, work in teams of three. Targets for their investigations are usually high-cost areas of medical or surgical practice. Table 7.2 summarizes some of the problems the groups have investigated. Each group provides a detailed, evidence-based set of three suggestions for how the problem might be addressed. The table shows the current cost of the problem, the strategies that might be used to address it, and the potential cost savings. A core assumption underlying these analyses is that the alternative strategies for managing these problems produce no harm for patients, are better aligned with patient and consumer preferences, and are derived from high-quality research evidence.

One example is care for late-stage cancer. Management of this phase of cancer is estimated to cost about $150 billion per year in the United States. It is often managed in the hospital. The Stanford analysis suggested that most patients prefer to be cared for at home, where they are near family and away from the sense of isolation that may occur in hospitals. The intervention strategies include better formulation of patient goals, effective use of pain management, and the application of treatments in the home or in facilities near the patient's residence. These programs were estimated to save approximately $37 billion per year.

Another example is stroke care. Currently, it is estimated that care for patients who have experienced a stroke costs about $48 billion per year nationally. Some patients experience unnecessary extra disability because the emergency response to the stroke is not optimal. Patients lose approximately two million brain cells each minute following a stroke. Most patients benefit from rapid administration of medicines that break up blood clots. However, these drugs can be dangerous when the stroke is associated with bleeding rather than blood clotting. Because of this concern, a series of evaluative steps, including a CAT scan of the head, are required. The Stanford group spent considerable time examining the process of evaluation and concluded that it could be streamlined. This streamlined process is now used by Kaiser Permanente in Northern California and is being evaluated for wider-scale application in Contra Costa, California. In addition to more rapid responses to strokes, the team recommended that some hospital care for stroke victims be replaced with high-quality home care and that medical groups use nurses to increase adherence to medicines that may protect adults who are at risk for stroke. It was estimated that these efforts would save about $2.8 billion per year.

A final example is critical care delivered in the intensive care unit (ICU). ICU care accounts for nearly three-quarters of 1 percent of the GDP in the United States. Other countries spend significantly less on intensive treatment, but often achieve better patient outcomes. In investigating the problem, the Stanford fellows learned from intensive care unit directors that as many as 40 percent of the patients in ICUs may not be sick enough to require care in a unit that assigns at least one full-time nurse to each patient. Another 25 percent of patients in ICUs may be so severely ill that medical care has little to offer them. The goal of this evaluation was to propose methods to care for seriously ill patients who may not benefit from being in the ICU. The fellows proposed using modern technologies to monitor patients in less staff-intensive areas of the hospital, with the opportunity for rapid transfer if a problem develops. In addition, they suggested evaluations that might reduce unnecessary ICU admissions, which may account for 65 percent of people currently being cared for in intensive care units. The analysis suggested that these policies, conservatively, could save about $42 billion per year.

The analyses by Berwick and Hackbarth and by the Stanford fellows clarify where the money to support a health System 3.0 might come from. Investing in behavioral and social determinants of health will cost money, but a new system may actually spend significantly less to achieve a healthier population. Reallocation decisions are always hard, yet we do have good evidence-based guidance on how to achieve more with less.

Conclusion

Our expensive and inefficient health care system must be redesigned to align with evidence concerning the factors associated with good health outcomes. Although this problem is underresearched, we do know that the narrow biomedical approach omits much that is important to longevity and quality of life. Helping well-insured people avoid illness through the modification of biological risk factors is useful, but it can't be all that we are good at. The need to account for all-cause mortality and social and behavioral determinants of health is widely recognized, but we still face a disconnect between understanding the problem and providing proposals for realistic solutions. Not that scientists, health providers, activists, and others don't have good ideas for doing better, but the major institutions tasked with ensuring public health have not caught up to the degree that is needed.

The United States has developed a health care system that is expert in the use of biomedicine. Our providers are enviably capable when it comes to helping sick patients, as long as those patients are able to afford the enormous cost of good care and as long as the pathologies of the system don't undermine its considerable capacities. But we have done too little to improve social and environmental conditions that mass-produce ill health in the first place.

To some extent, improvement can happen at the receiving end of the system, where doctors treat patients. But we ought to start with science. We should continue doing biomedical science, but in the context of a truly multidisciplinary research agenda. Creating efficient pathways to wellness requires new priorities. It requires not more spending but different spending. And, reasonable, evidence-based blueprints already exist for how money can be saved and redeployed for the common purpose of enhancing health. Ultimately, changing the way we seek to improve health will bring savings in the form of greater wellness and lower health care costs. There is plenty of work to do.

Appendix

Notes

Acknowledgments

Credits

Index

appendix

Behavior-Health Linkages among Major
"Actual Causes" of Death and Major Diseases

Linkage 1—Behavioral, Environmental, and Genetic
Influences Moderate One Another

TOBACCO USE Both environmental and genetic factors influence onset and persistence of smoking.[1]

DIET Studies of food preferences indicate genetic influences are smaller than environmental influences.[2]

PHYSICAL ACTIVITY Twin studies find that, even among genetically high-risk individuals, greater physical activity levels are associated with lower rates of obesity.[3]

ALCOHOL USE Childhood maltreatment exacerbates genetic influences on adult alcohol use and antisocial personality among women and men.[4]

CARDIOVASCULAR DISEASE AND DIABETES Influence of serotonin transporter gene on cardiovascular risk is moderated by stress and environmental factors.[5]

CANCER Nutrition and lifestyle intervention reduce prostate gene expression and tumorigenesis in men.[6]

HIV/AIDS In monkey models of HIV, individual characteristics (sociability), stable versus unstable social conditions, and genotype for the serotonin transporter gene interact in affecting disease progression.[7]

Linkage 2—Behavior Influences Health

TOBACCO USE Numerous surgeon general's reports have concluded that smoking is a leading cause of cancer, cardiovascular and pulmonary disease, and premature death.[8]

DIET Systematic reviews conclude that obesity contributes to hypertension, hyperlipidemia, diabetes, cardiovascular disease, and some cancers.[9]

PHYSICAL ACTIVITY Randomized trials and systematic reviews conclude that physical activity is associated with decreased all-cause mortality[10] and reduced incidence of chronic diseases and breast cancer, specifically.[11]

ALCOHOL USE Alcohol abuse itself is associated with motor vehicle crashes, homicides, suicides, and drowning. Long-term heavy drinking can lead to heart disease, cancer, alcohol-related liver disease, and pancreatitis. Alcohol use during pregnancy is known to cause fetal alcohol syndrome, a leading cause of preventable mental retardation.[12]

CARDIOVASCULAR DISEASE AND DIABETES Diet and obesity are risk factors for diabetes and cardiovascular disease.[13]

CANCER Findings from systematic reviews, meta-analyses, large prospective studies, and randomized trials link cancer risk with poor diet, physical inactivity, smoking, stress, and social involvement.[14]

HIV/AIDS Substantial and consistent evidence shows that chronic depression, stressful events, and trauma may negatively affect HIV disease progression.[15]

Linkage 3—Behavior Change Interventions Prevent Disease

TOBACCO USE A major multisite trial demonstrated that smoking cessation programs substantially reduce mortality even when only a minority of patients stop smoking.[16]

DIET Systematic reviews and randomized trials show that childhood dietary interventions have positive impacts on weight-gain trajectory, weight-loss maintenance,[17] and insulin resistance.[18]

PHYSICAL ACTIVITY Among overweight, previously inactive women at risk for type 2 diabetes, accumulating 10,000 steps/day for eight weeks improved glucose tolerance and reduced both systolic and diastolic blood pressure.[19]

ALCOHOL USE Among pregnant women, fifteen minutes of counseling increased abstinence from drinking by five times relative to controls and resulted in higher birth weights and birth lengths. Fetal mortality was reduced threefold, from 2.9 percent to 0.9 percent.[20]

CARDIOVASCULAR DISEASE AND DIABETES Lifestyle interventions focusing on diet, weight loss, and exercise can reduce incidence of diabetes among people at risk for the disease.[21]

CANCER A number of large prospective longitudinal studies and meta-analyses link physical activity to reduced risk of colon cancer.[22]

HIV/AIDS The US Preventive Services Task Force recommends high-intensity behavioral counseling to prevent sexually transmitted infections for all sexually active adolescents and for adults at heightened risk.[23]

Linkage 4—Behavior Change Interventions Improve Disease Management

TOBACCO USE Self-management skills (e.g., setting a quit date, planning to cope with cravings) help people quit smoking.[24]

DIET Randomized behavioral interventions show that peer nutrition education positively influences diabetes self-management in Latinos.[25]

PHYSICAL ACTIVITY Randomized clinical trials show that exercise training reduces levels of glycated hemoglobin among those with diabetes.[26]

ALCOHOL USE Brief counseling sessions with follow-up produce small to moderate reductions in alcohol consumption, sustained for six months or longer.[27]

CARDIOVASCULAR DISEASE AND DIABETES Diabetes self-management programs improve disease management[28] and metabolic control,[29] including among older adults and ethnic minorities,[30] and reduce complications[31] as well as incidence of heart attack, stroke, and death from cardiovascular disease.[32]

Interventions promoting comprehensive lifestyle changes for patients with coronary artery disease can reduce progression of coronary atherosclerosis and incidence of cardiac events,[33] encourage smoking cessation, improve functional capacity, lower LDL cholesterol, and reduce all-cause mortality.[34]

CANCER Randomized trials of patients with cancer indicate that physical activity increases functional capacity during chemotherapy, improves bone marrow recovery and decreases complications during peripheral blood stem transplantation, and reduces the burden of symptoms associated with radiation therapy and chemotherapy, such as fatigue.[35]

HIV/AIDS Behavioral interventions have improved adherence to medication plans and disease management generally.[36]

Linkage 5—Psychosocial and Behavioral Interventions Improve Quality of Life

TOBACCO USE Ex-smokers have significantly improved quality of life compared with current smokers.[37]

DIET In randomized trials, individuals who experienced lifestyle interventions had improved nutritional status and physical functioning less depressive symptoms.[38]

PHYSICAL ACTIVITY Randomized trials show physical activity improves quality of life among, for instance, older adults.[39] Exercise also improves quality of life and reduces fatigue among breast cancer survivors.[40]

ALCOHOL USE Cognitive-behavioral treatment among recovering alcoholics improved measures of sleep, depression, anxiety, and quality of life.[41]

CARDIOVASCULAR DISEASE AND DIABETES Among patients with cardiovascular disease or diabetes, comprehensive behavioral disease-management interventions improve a variety of clinical indicators and reduce general distress and depressive symptoms,[42] improve emotional and social functioning,[43] reduce anxiety,[44] and improve overall quality of life.[45]

CANCER Randomized psychosocial interventions are associated with decreased psychological distress, less pain and nausea incident to treatment, and improved immune-system modulation and quality of life.[46]

HIV/AIDS Stress-management interventions enhance emotional status and quality of life.[47]

Linkage 6—Health Promotion Programs Improve Health of Populations

TOBACCO USE A California anti-smoking campaign involving counter-media, youth prevention programs, cessation services, and tax increases reduced smoking, rates of cardiovascular disease,[48] and death rates from lung cancer.[49]

DIET Health education campaigns[50] and policy and environmental supports[51] can lead to significant dietary improvements in the general population.

PHYSICAL ACTIVITY Walk-to-school programs increase walking and biking to school. Providing walking and fitness trails has been shown to increase physical activity in an at-risk population.[52]

ALCOHOL USE Regulating the density of alcohol sellers within communities reduces consumption, and enforcing prohibitions of sales to minors reduces underage consumption.[53]

Source: Reformatted from Edwin B. Fisher, Marian L. Fitzgibbon, Russell E. Glasgow, et al., "Behavior Matters," *American Journal of Preventive Medicine* 40, no. 5 (2011), table 1.

notes

Abbreviations

JAMA: Journal of the American Medical Association
NEJM: New England Journal of Medicine
PNAS: Proceedings of the National Academy of Sciences

Introduction

1. E. J. Emanuel, "How Can the United States Spend Its Health Care Dollars Better?" *JAMA* 316 (2016): 2604–2606.
2. Francis S. Collins, "Testimony on the Fiscal Year 2012 Budget Request before the Senate Committee," National Institutes of Health, May 10, 2011, https://www.nih.gov/about-nih/who-we-are/nih-director/fiscal-year-2012-budget-request-senate.
3. M. J. Joyner, N. Paneth, and J. P. A. Ioannidis, "What Happens When Underperforming Big Ideas in Research Become Entrenched?" *JAMA* 316, no. 13 (2016): 1355–1356.
4. A. Case and A. Deaton, "Rising Morbidity and Mortality in Midlife among White Non-Hispanic Americans in the 21st Century," *PNAS* 112, no. 49 (2015): 15078–15083.
5. S. H. Woolf and L. Y. Aron, "The US Health Disadvantage Relative to Other High-Income Countries: Findings from a National Research Council / Institute of Medicine Report," *JAMA* 309 (2013): 771–772.
6. S. H. Woolf, "The Big Answer: Rediscovering Prevention at a Time of Crisis in Health Care," *Harvard Health Policy Review* 7 (2006): 5–20.
7. A. Fenelon and S. H. Preston, "Estimating Smoking-Attributable Mortality in the United States," *Demography* 49 (2012): 797–818.
8. D. D. Abrams, A. M. Glasser, A. C. Villanti, and R. Niaura, "Cigarettes: The Rise and Decline but not Demise of the Greatest Behavioral Health Disaster of the 20th Century," in *Population Health: Behavioral and Social Science Insights,* ed. R. M. Kaplan, M. L. Spittel, and D. H. David (Rockville, MD: Agency for Healthcare Research and Quality and Office of Behavioral and Social Sciences Research, National Institutes of Health, 2015), 143–168.
9. R. M. Kaplan and V. L. Irvin, "Likelihood of Null Effects of Large NHLBI Clinical Trials Has Increased over Time," *PLOS One* 10 (2015): e0132382.
10. P. Kellner, "Do Britons Understand the U.S. Better than Americans?" YouGov, January 25, 2013, https://today.yougov.com/topics/politics/articles-reports/2013/01/25/do-britons-understand-us-better-americans.
11. C. E. Steuerle, *Dead Men Ruling: How to Restore Fiscal Freedom and Rescue Our Future* (New York: Century Foundation Press, 2014).

12. E. H. Bradley, B. R. Elkins, J. Herrin, and B. Elbel, "Health and Social Services Expenditures: Associations with Health Outcomes," *BMJ Quality and Safety* 20 (2011): 826–831.

13. A. L. Kellermann and F. P. Rivara, "Silencing the Science on Gun Research," *JAMA* 309 (2013): 549–550.

1. Let's Be Average

1. V. Bush, *Science: The Endless Frontier* (Washington, DC: Office of Scientific Research and Development, 1945).

2. V .R. Fuchs, "Social Determinants of Health: Caveats and Nuances," *JAMA* 317 (2017): 25–26.

3. Fuchs, "Social Determinants of Health," 25–26.

4. D. A. Kindig and E. R. Cheng, "Even as Mortality Fell in Most US Counties, Female Mortality Nonetheless Rose in 42.8 Percent of Counties from 1992 to 2006," *Health Affairs* 32 (2013): 451–458; A. Case and A. Deaton, "Rising Morbidity and Mortality," in Midlife among White Non-Hispanic Americans in the 21st Century," *PNAS* 112 (2015): 15078–15083. Even as mortality fell in most US counties, female mortality nonetheless rose in 42.8 percent of counties from 1992 to 2006.

5. The name of the Istitution of Medicine changed to National Academy of Medicine in 2015.

6. Institute of Medicine, *For the Public's Health: Investing in a Healthier Future* (Washington, DC: National Academies Press, 2012).

7. U. E. Reinhardt, P. S. Hussey, and G .F. Anderson, "U.S. Health Care Spending in an International Context," *Health Affairs* 23 (2004): 10–25.

8. E. M. Crimmins, S. H. Preston, and B. Cohen, *Explaining Divergent Levels of Longevity in High-Income Countries* (Washington, DC: National Academies Press, 2011).

9. S. H. Woolf and L. Aron, eds., *US Health in International Perspective: Shorter Lives, Poorer Health* (Washington, DC: National Academies Press, 2013).

10. M. L. Conte, J. Liu, S. Schnell, and M. B. Omary, "Globalization and Changing Trends of Biomedical Research Output," *JCI Insight* 2, no. 12 (2017): e95206.

11. P. R. Orszag, "How Health Care Can Save or Sink America: The Case for Reform and Fiscal Sustainability," *Foreign Affairs* 90 (2011): 42.

12. Tom Epstein, "Republicans Should Focus on Health Care Issues That Matter, like Skyrocketing Costs," *Sacramento Bee,* December 29, 2016, http://www .sacbee.com/opinion/article123486264.html.

13. D. M. Cutler and M. McClellan, "Is Technological Change in Medicine Worth It?," *Health Affairs* 20, no. 5 (2001): 11–29.

14. D. M. Cutler, A. B. Rosen, and S. Vijan, "The Value of Medical Spending in the United States, 1960–2000," *NEJM* 355 (2006): 920–927.

15. L. Goldman and E. F. Cook, "The Decline in Ischemic Heart Disease Mortality Rates: An Analysis of the Comparative Effects of Medical Interventions and Changes in Lifestyle," *Annals of Internal Medicine* 101 (1984): 825–836; B. Unal, J. A. Critchley, and S. Capewell, "Explaining the Decline in Coronary

Heart Disease Mortality in England and Wales between 1981 and 2000," *Circulation* 109 (2004): 1101–1107.

16. R. M. Kaplan, "Behavior Change and Reducing Health Disparities," *Preventive Medicine* 68 (2014): 5–10; S. A. Schroeder, "We Can Do Better—Improving the Health of the American People," *NEJM* 357 (2007): 1221–1228; D. E. Wennberg, S. M. Sharp, G. Bevan, et al., "A Population Health Approach to Reducing Observational Intensity Bias in Health Risk Adjustment: Cross Sectional Analysis of Insurance Claims," *BMJ* 348 (2014): g2392.

17. D. C. Goodman, E. S. Fisher, G. A. Little, et al., "The Relation between the Availability of Neonatal Intensive Care and Neonatal Mortality," *NEJM* 346 (2002): 1538–1544.

18. "The World: Infant Mortality Rate (2016)—Top 100+," http://www.geoba.se /population.php?pc=world&type=019&year=2016&st.

19. R. M. Kaplan, "Variation between End-of-Life Health Care Costs in Los Angeles and San Diego: Why Are They So Different?" *Journal of Palliative Medicine* 14 (2011): 215–220.

20. E. S. Fisher, D. E. Wennberg, T. A. Stukel, et al., "The Implications of Regional Variations in Medicare Spending, Part 2: Health Outcomes and Satisfaction with Care," *Annals of Internal Medicine* 138 (2003): 288–298.

21. J. E. Wennberg, J. L. Freeman, and W. J. Culp, "Are Hospital Services Rationed in New Haven or Over-Utilised in Boston?" *Lancet* 329, no. 8543 (1987): 1185–1189.

22. J. E. Wennberg, "Forty Years of Unwarranted Variation—And Still Counting," *Health Policy* 114, no. 1 (2014): 1–2; J. Busby, S. Purdy, and W. Hollingworth, "A Systematic Review of the Magnitude and Cause of Geographic Variation in Unplanned Hospital Admission Rates and Length of Stay for Ambulatory Care Sensitive Conditions," *BMC Health Services Research* 15 (2015).

23. J. E. Wennberg, "Small Area Analysis and the Medical Care Outcome Problem," in *Research Methodology: Strengthening Causal Interpretations of Nonexperimental Data,* ed. L. Sechrest, E. Perrin, and J. Bunker (Rockville, MD: Department of Health and Human Services, Agency for Health Care Policy and Research, 1990), 177–206.

24. World Health Organization (WHO), *Global Health Risks—Mortality and Burden of Disease Attributable to Selected Major Risks,* October 28, 2009, http://www.thehealthwell.info/node/9612.

25. S. Kumar and A. S. Kelly, "Review of Childhood Obesity: From Epidemiology, Etiology, and Comorbidities to Clinical Assessment and Treatment," *Mayo Clinic Proceedings* 92, no. 2 (2017): 251–265.

26. G. S. Yeo, "Genetics of Obesity: Can an Old Dog Teach Us New Tricks?" *Diabetologia* 60 (2017): 778–783; J. Lakerveld and J. Mackenbach, "The Upstream Determinants of Adult Obesity," *Obesity Facts* 10 (2017): 216–222.

27. K. Silventoinen, A. Jelenkovic, R. Sund, et al., "Genetic and Environmental Effects on Body Mass Index from Infancy to the Onset of Adulthood: An Individual-Based Pooled Analysis of 45 Twin Cohorts Participating in the Collaborative Project of Development of Anthropometrical Measures in Twins (CODATwins) Study," *American Journal of Clinical Nutrition* 104 (2016): 371–379.

28. W. H. Dietz, B. Belay, D. Bradley, et al., "A Model Framework That Integrates Community and Clinical Systems for the Prevention and Management of Obesity and Other Chronic Diseases," Discussion Paper, National Academy of Medicine, January 13, 2017.

29. S. Gallus, A. Lugo, B. Murisic, et al., "Overweight and Obesity in 16 European Countries," *European Journal of Nutrition* 54 (2015): 679–689.

30. S. Lisonkova, J. Potts, G. M. Muraca, N. Razaz, Y. Sabr, and W.-S. Chan, "588: The Effect of Maternal Age on Severe Maternal Morbidity and Perinatal Outcomes," *American Journal of Obstetrics and Gynecology* 216, no. 1 (2017): S347.

31. World Health Organization (WHO), *Global Health Risks—Mortality and Burden of Disease Attributable to Selected Major Risks.*

32. Case and Deaton, "Rising Morbidity and Mortality."

33. "Prescription Opiod Overdose Data," Centers for Disease Control and Prevention, https://www.cdc.gov/drugoverdose/data/overdose.html.

34. Case and Deaton, "Rising Morbidity and Mortality," 15078–15083.

35. N. Kristof, "How to Win a War on Drugs," *New York Times,* September 22, 2017.

36. Kindig and Cheng, "Even as Mortality Fell in Most US Counties, Female Mortality Nonetheless Rose in 42.8 Percent of Counties from 1992 to 2006," 451–458.

37. R. M. Kaplan, Z. Fang, and J. Kirby, "Educational Attainment and Health Outcomes: Data from the Medical Expenditures Panel Survey," *Health Psychology* 36, no. 6 (2017): 598–608.

38. J. C. Wright and M. C. Weinstein, "Gains in Life Expectancy from Medical Interventions—Standardizing Data on Outcomes," *NEJM* 339 (1998): 380–386.

39. Woolf and Aron, *US Health in International Perspective.*

40. V. R. Fuchs and A. Milstein, "The $640 Billion Question—Why Does Cost-Effective Care Diffuse So Slowly?" *NEJM* 364 (2011): 1985–1987.

2. Research Promise and Practice

1. "NIADI Budget Data Comparisons," *National Institute for Allergies and Infectious Diseases,* https://www.niaid.nih.gov/grants-contracts/niaid-budget-data-comparisons.

2. T. Maughan, "The Promise and the Hype of 'Personalised Medicine,'" *New Bioethics* 23, no. 1 (2017): 13–20.

3. J. C. Venter, *A Life Decoded: My Genome, My Life* (New York: Penguin 2007).

4. N. Wade, "A Decade Later, Genetic Map Yields Few New Cures," *New York Times,* June 13, 2010, http://www.nytimes.com/2010/06/13/health/research/13genome.html.

5. T. Caulfield, "Genetics and Personalized Medicine: Where's the Revolution?" blog post, *BMJ Clinical Evidence,* July 23, 2015, https://blogs.bmj.com/bmj/2015/07/23/timothy-caulfield-genetics-and-personalized-medicine-wheres-the-revolution/.

6. S. L. Ginn, I. E. Alexander, M. L. Edelstein, et al., "Gene Therapy Clinical Trials Worldwide to 2012—An Update," *Journal of Gene Medicine* 15 (2013): 65–77.

7. N. P. Paynter, D. I. Chasman, G. Pare, et al., "Association between a Literature-Based Genetic Risk Score and Cardiovascular Events in Women," *JAMA* 303, no. 7 (2010): 631–637.

8. E. J. Benjamin, M. J. Blaha, S. E. Chiuve, et al., "Heart Disease and Stroke Statistics—2017 Update: A Report from the American Heart Association," *Circulation* 135, no. 10 (2017):e146–e603.

9. L. A. Miosge, M. A. Field, Y. Sontani, et al., "Comparison of Predicted and Actual Consequences of Missense Mutations," *PNAS* 112, no. 37 (2015): E5189–E5198.

10. M. J. Joyner, "'Moonshot' Medicine Will Let Us Down," *New York Times,* January 29, 2015.

11. M. A. Andersson, S. K. Gadarian, and R. Almeling, "Does Educational Attainment Shape Reactions to Genetic Risk for Alzheimer's Disease? Results from a National Survey Experiment," *Social Science and Medicine* 180 (2017): 101–105; E. A Waters, L. Ball, and S. Gehlert, "'I Don't Believe It': Acceptance and Skepticism of Genetic Health Information among African-American and White Smokers," *Social Science and Medicine* 184 (2017): 153–160.

12. R. M. Kaplan, "Behavior Change and Reducing Health Disparities," *Preventive Medicine* 68 (2014): 5–10.

13. US Food and Drug Administration, *The Public Health Evidence for FDA Oversight of Laboratory Developed Tests: 20 Studies* (Silver Spring, MD: US Food and Drug Administration, 2015).

14. US Food and Drug Administration, *The Public Health Evidence for FDA Oversight of Laboratory Developed Tests.*

15. J. Hicks and A. Krasnitz, "Genetic Markers Indicative of a Cancer Patient Response to Trastuzumab (Herceptin)," US Patent 9677139B2, filed June 7, 2012, and issued June 13, 2017.

16. J. Gill, A. J. Obley, and V. Prasad, "Direct-to-Consumer Genetic Testing: The Implications of the US FDA's First Marketing Authorization for BRCA Mutation Testing," *JAMA* 319 (2018): 2377–2378.

17. P. K. Chaitanya, K. A. Kumar, B. Stalin, et al., "The Role of Mutation Testing in Patients with Chronic Myeloid Leukemia in Chronic Phase after Imatinib Failure and Their Outcomes after Treatment Modification: Single-Institutional Experience over 13 years," *Indian Journal of Medical and Paediatric Oncology* 38 (2017): 328–333.

18. S. S. Ning Tan, A. Y. Yip Fong, M. Mejin, et al., "Association of *CYP2C19*2* Polymorphism with Clopidogrel Response and 1-Year Major Adverse Cardiovascular Events in a Multiethnic Population with Drug-Eluting Stents," *Pharmacogenomics* 18, no. 13 (2017): 1225–1239.

19. K. Stergiopoulos and D. L. Brown, "Genotype-Guided vs. Clinical Dosing of Warfarin and its Analogues: Meta-Analysis of Randomized Clinical Trials," *JAMA Internal Medicine* 174 (2014): 1330–1338.

20. R. K. Friedman, "Infidelity Lurks in Your Genes," *New York Times,* May 22, 2015.

21. T. R. Insel, "The Challenge of Translation in Social Neuroscience: A Review of Oxytocin, Vasopressin, and Affiliative Behavior," *Neuron* 65 (2010): 768–779.

22. Insel, "The Challenge of Translation," 768–779.

23. W. Simon, *Sexual Conduct: The Social Sources of Human Sexuality* (Abingdon: Routledge, 2017).

24. H. Walum, L. Westberg, S. Henningsson, et al., "Genetic Variation in the Vasopressin Receptor 1a Gene (AVPR1A) Associates with Pair-Bonding Behavior in Humans," *PNAS* 105 (2008): 14153–14156.

25. D. G. Mitchem, B. P. Zietsch, M. J. Wright, et al., "No Relationship between Intelligence and Facial Attractiveness in a Large, Genetically Informative Sample," *Evolution and Human Behavior* 36 (2015): 240–247.

26. F. S. Collins and H. Varmus, "A New Initiative on Precision Medicine," *NEJM* 372 (2015): 793–795.

27. S. D. Shapiro, "The Promise of Precision Medicine for Health Systems," *American Journal of Health-System Pharmacy* 73 (2016) 1907–1908.

28. E. A. Ashley, "The Precision Medicine Initiative: A New National Effort," *JAMA* 313 (2015): 2119–2120.

29. C. Neti, S. Ebadollahi, M. Kohn, and D. Ferrucci, "'IBM Watson + Data Analytics': A Big Data Analytics Approach for a Learning Healthcare System," *IEEE eNewsletter,* May 2012, http://lifesciences.ieee.org/lifesciences -newsletter/2012/may-2012/ibm-watson-data-analytics-a-big-data-analytics -approach-for-a-learning-healthcare-system/.

30. G. B. Mills, "Delivering on the Promise of Personalized Medicine," *Clinical Cancer Research* 22, no. 1, suppl. (2016), abstract nr IA17.

31. M. J. Khoury and S. Galea, "Will Precision Medicine Improve Population Health?" *JAMA* 316 (2016): 1357–1358.

32. M. R. Tonelli and B. H. Shirts, "Knowledge for Precision Medicine: Mechanistic Reasoning and Methodological Pluralism," *JAMA* 318, no. 17 (2017): 1649–1650.

33. T. Caulfield, D. Sipp, C. E. Murry, et al., "Confronting Stem Cell Hype," *Science* 352 (2016): 776–777.

34. M. J. Joyner, N. Paneth, and J. P. Ioannidis, "What Happens When Underper-forming Big Ideas in Research Become Entrenched?" *JAMA* 316, no. 13 (2016): 1335–1356.

35. R. Horton, "Offline: What Is Medicine's 5 Sigma?" *Lancet* 385 (2015): 1380.

36. J. P. Ioannidis, "Why Most Published Research Findings Are False," *PLOS Medicine* 2, no. 8 (2005): e124.

37. B. D. Earp and D. Wilkinson, "The Publication Symmetry Test: A Simple Editorial Heuristic to Combat Publication Bias," *Journal of Clinical and Transitional Research* 3 (2017): 5–7.

38. J. P. Ioannidis "Why Most Clinical Research Is Not Useful," *PLOS Medicine* 13 (2016): e1002049.

39. R. Chatterjee, "Cases of Mistaken Identity," *Science* 315 (2007): 928.

40. J. L. Cummings, T. Morstorf, and K. Zhong, "Alzheimer's Disease Drug-Development Pipeline: Few Candidates, Frequent Failures," *Alzheimers Research and Therapy* 6 (2014): 37.

41. N. Weiner, *Cybernetics: Or, Control and Communication in the Animal and in the Machine* (Cambridge, MA: MIT Press, 1948).

42. M. Lauer, "A Look at NIH Support for Model Organisms, Part Two," NIH *Extramural Nexus,* Open Mike blog post, August 3, 2016, https://nexus.od.nih .gov/all/2016/08/03/model-organisms-part-two/.

43. "How Science Goes Wrong," *Economist,* October, 21, 2013, https://www .economist.com/news/leaders/21588069-scientific-research-has-changed-world -now-it-needs-change-itself-how-science-goes-wrong; "Trouble at the Lab," *Economist,* October 18, 2013, https://www.economist.com/news/briefing /21588057-scientists-think-science-self-correcting-alarming-degree-it-not-trouble.

44. L. P. Freedman, I. M. Cockbur, and T. S. Simcoe, "The Economics of Reproducibility in Preclinical Research," *PLOS Biology* 13, no. 6 (2015): e1002165.

45. B. A. Nosek and T. M. Errington, "Reproducibility in Cancer Biology: Making Sense of Replications," *eLife* 6 (2017): e23383.

46. F. Prinz, T. Schlange, and K. Asadullah, "Believe It or Not: How Much Can We Rely on Published Data on Potential Drug Targets? *Nature Reviews: Drug Discovery* 10, no. 9 (2011): 712.

47. Prinz, Schlange, and Asadullah, "Believe It or Not."

48. F. S. Collins and L. A. Tabak, "Policy: NIH Plans to Enhance Reproducibility," *Nature* 505 (2014): 612–613.

49. B. T. Gehr, C. Weiss, and F. Porzsolt, "The Fading of Reported Effectiveness: A Meta-Analysis of Randomised Controlled Trials," *BMC Medical Research Methodology* 6, no. 1 (2006): 25; J. Schooler, "Unpublished Results Hide the Decline Effect," *Nature* 470 (2011): 437.

50. D. A. Chambers, "Advancing Sustainability Research: Challenging Existing Paradigms," *Journal of Public Health Dentistry* 71, suppl. 1 (2011): S99–100.

51. J. Anomaly, "Ethics, Antibiotics, and Public Policy," *Georgetown Journal of Law and Public Policy* 15 (2017): 999–1015.

52. L. W. Green, J. Ottoson, C. Garcia, et al., "Diffusion Theory and Knowledge Dissemination, Utilization, and Integration in Public Health," *Annual Review of Public Health* 30 (2009): 151–174.

53. G. Neta, R. E. Glasgow, C. R. Carpenter, et al., "A Framework for Enhancing the Value of Research for Dissemination and Implementation," *American Journal of Public Health* 105 (2015): 49–57.

54. R. E. Glasgow, C. Vinson, D. Chambers, et al., "National Institutes of Health Approaches to Dissemination and Implementation Science: Current and Future Directions," *American Journal of Public Health* 102 (2012): 1274–1281.

55. F. Gueyffier, C. Bulpitt, J. P. Boissel, et al., "Antihypertensive Drugs in Very Old People: A Subgroup Meta-Analysis of Randomised Controlled Trials," *Lancet* 353 (1999): 793–796.

56. R. F. Redberg and M. H. Katz, "Statins for Primary Prevention: The Debate Is Intense, but the Data Are Weak," *JAMA Internal Medicine* 177 (2017): 21–23.

57. J. H. Mieres, M. Gulati, N. Bairey Merz, et al., "Role of Noninvasive Testing in the Clinical Evaluation of Women with Suspected Ischemic Heart Disease: A Consensus Statement from the American Heart Association," *Circulation* 130 (2014): 350–379; R. F. Redberg, "Don't Assume Women Are the Same as Men: Include Them in the Trial," *Archives of Internal Medicine* 172 (2012): 921.

58. R. M. Kaplan and V. L. Irvin, "Likelihood of Null Effects of Large NHLBI Clinical Trials Has Increased over Time," *PlOS One* 10 (2015): e0132382.

59. A. Bowen and A. Casadevall, "Increasing Disparities between Resource Inputs and Outcomes, as Measured by Certain Health Deliverables, in Biomedical Research," *PNAS* 112, no. 36 (2015): 11335–11340.

60. J. Watson, *The Double Helix: The Discovery of the Structure of DNA* (London: Hachette, 2012); J. D. Watson and F. H. Crick, "Molecular Structure of Nucleic Acids," *Nature* 171 (1953): 737–738.

61. S. Theil, "Trouble in Mind," *Scientific American* 313 (2015): 36–42.

62. Theil, "Trouble in Mind."

63. J. M. Perrin, S. P. Batlivala, and T. L. Cheng, "In the Aftermath of the National Children's Study," *JAMA Pediatrics* 169 (2015): 519–520.

64. J. Kaiser, "NIH Puts Massive US Children's Study on Hold," *Science* 344 (2014): 1327.

65. N. Bloom, C. I. Jones, J. Van Reenen, and M. Webb, "Are Ideas Getting Harder to Find?" NBER working paper no. 23782, September 2017, http://www.nber .org/papers/w23782.

66. A. Rogers, "Star Neuroscientist Tom Insel Leaves the Google-Spawned Verily for . . . A Startup?" *Wired,* June 11, 2017, https://www.wired.com/2017/05/star -neuroscientist-tom-insel-leaves-google-spawned-verily-startup/.

3. Mistaking the Meaning of Health

1. R. E. Schoen, P. F. Pinsky, J. L. Weissfeld, et al., "Colorectal-Cancer Incidence and Mortality with Screening Flexible Sigmoidoscopy," *NEJM* 366 (2012): 2345–2357.

2. J. S. Lin, M. A. Piper, L. A. Perdue, et al., "Screening for Colorectal Cancer: Updated Evidence Report and Systematic Review for the US Preventive Services Task Force," *JAMA* 315 (2016): 2576–2594.

3. J. S. Mandel, T. R. Church, F. Ederer, and J. H. Bond, "Colorectal Cancer Mortality: Effectiveness of Biennial Screening for Fecal Occult Blood," *Journal of the National Cancer Institute* 91 (1999): 434–437.

4. P. A. Ubel, "Medical Facts versus Value Judgments—Toward Preference-Sensitive Guidelines," *NEJM* 372 (2015): 2475–2477; P. A. Ubel, D. A. Comerford, and E. Johnson, "Healthcare.gov 3.0—Behavioral Economics and Insurance Exchanges," *NEJM* 372 (2015): 695–698; M. Roland and R. A. Dudley, "How Financial and Reputational Incentives Can Be Used to Improve Medical Care," *Health Services Research Journal* 50, no. S2 (2015): 2090–2115.

5. R. M. Kaplan, "The Ziggy Theorem: Toward an Outcomes-Focused Health Psychology," *Health Psychology* 13, no. 6 (1994): 451–460; "Better Care. Smarter Spending. Healthier People: Paying Providers for Value, Not Volume," fact sheet, Centers for Medicare and Medicaid Services, January 26, 2015, https://www.cms.gov/Newsroom/MediaReleaseDatabase/Fact-sheets/2015-Fact -sheets-items/2015-01-26-3.html.

6. R. M. Kaplan and J. P. Anderson, "A General Health Policy Model: Update and Applications," *Health Services Research* 23 (1988): 203–235.

7. D. G. Fryback, N. C. Dunham, M. Palta, et al., "US Norms for Six Generic Health-Related Quality-of-Life Indexes from the National Health Measurement Study," *Medical Care* 45 (2007): 1162–1170; R. M. Kaplan, S. Tally, R. D. Hays, et al., "Five Preference-Based Indexes in Cataract and Heart Failure Patients Were Not Equally Responsive to Change," *Journal of Clinical Epidemiology* 64 (2011): 497–506.

8. D. B. Abrams, "Applying Transdisciplinary Research Strategies to Understanding and Eliminating Health Disparities," *Health Education and Behavior* 33, no. 4 (2006): 515–531; R. M. Kaplan, "The Future of Outcomes Measurement in Rheumatology," *American Journal of Managed Care* 13, no. 9, suppl. (2007): S252–S255; R. M. Kaplan and D. L. Frosch, "Decision Making in Medicine and Health Care," *Annual Review of Clinical Psychology* 1 (2005): 525–556; R. M. Kaplan and A. L. Ries, "Quality of Life: Concept and Definition," *Journal of Chronic Obstructive Pulmonary Disease* 4, no. 3 (2007): 263–271.

9. "Know Your Health Numbers," American Heart Association, http://www.heart .org/HEARTORG/Conditions/More/Diabetes/PreventionTreatmentofDiabetes /Know-Your-Health-Numbers_UCM_313882_Article.jsp#.WsV6RYjwY2w.

10. "Framingham Coronary Heart Disease Risk Score," MDCalc, https://www .mdcalc.com/framingham-coronary-heart-disease-risk-score.

11. K. C. Stange and R. L. Ferrer, "The Paradox of Primary Care," *Annals of Family Medicine* 7 (2009): 293–299.

12. F. E. Young, S. L. Nightingale, and R. A. Temple, "The Preliminary Report of the Findings of the Aspirin Component of the Ongoing Physicians' Health Study: The FDA Perspective on Aspirin for the Primary Prevention of Myocardial Infarction," *JAMA* 259 (1988): 3158–3160.

13. R. M. Kaplan, "Health Outcome Models for Policy Analysis," *Health Psychology* 8 (1989): 723–735.

14. Action to Control Cardiovascular Risk in Diabetes Study Group, "Effects of Intensive Glucose Lowering in Type 2 Diabetes," *NEJM* 358 (2008): 2545–2559.

15. Action to Control Cardiovascular Risk in Diabetes Study Group, "Effects of Intensive Glucose Lowering."

16. J. B. Green, M. A. Bethel, P. W. Armstrong, et al., "Effect of Sitagliptin on Cardiovascular Outcomes in Type 2 Diabetes," *NEJM* 373 (2015): 232–242.

17. A. Qaseem, T. J. Wilt, D. Kansagara, et al., "Hemoglobin A1c Targets for Glycemic Control with Pharmacologic Therapy for Nonpregnant Adults with Type 2 Diabetes Mellitus: A Guidance Statement Update from the American College of Physicians," *Annals of Internal Medicine* 168, no. 8 (2018): 569–576.

18. T. B. Drüeke, F. Locatelli, N. Clyne, et al., "Normalization of Hemoglobin Level in Patients with Chronic Kidney Disease and Anemia," *NEJM* 355 (2006): 2071–2084.

19. T. Rupp and D. Zuckerman, "Quality of Life, Overall Survival, and Costs of Cancer Drugs Approved Based on Surrogate Endpoints," *JAMA Internal Medicine* 177, no. 2 (2017): 276–277.

20. The HPS2-Thrive Collaborative Group, "Effects of Extended-Release Niacin with Laropiprant in High-Risk Patients," *NEJM* 371 (2014): 203–212.

21. M. S. Sabatine, R. P. Giugliano, A. C. Keech, et al., "Evolocumab and Clinical Outcomes in Patients with Cardiovascular Disease," *NEJM* 376, no. 18 (2017): 1713–1722.

22. R. M. Kaplan and V. L. Irvin, "Likelihood of Null Effects of Large NHLBI Clinical Trials Has Increased over Time," *PLOS One* 10 (2015): e0132382.

23. S. R. Group, J. T. Wright Jr., J. D. Williamson, et al., "A Randomized Trial of Intensive versus Standard Blood-Pressure Control," *NEJM* 373 (2015): 2103–2116.

24. P. Muntner, R. M. Carey, S. Gidding, et al., "Potential U.S. Population Impact of the 2017 American College of Cardiology/American Heart Association High Blood Pressure Guideline," *Circulation* 71, no. 2 (2017): 109–118.

25. P. A. James, S. Oparil, B. L. Carter, et al., "2014 Evidence-Based Guideline for the Management of High Blood Pressure in Adults: Report from the Panel Members Appointed to the Eighth Joint National Committee (JNC 8)," *JAMA* 311 (2014): 507–520.

26. R. M. Kaplan and M. Ong, "Rationale and Public Health Implications of Changing CHD Risk Factor Definitions," *Annual Review of Public Health* 28 (2007): 321–344.

27. J. D. Bundy, K. T. Mills, J. Chen, et al., "Estimating the Association of the 2017 and 2014 Hypertension Guidelines with Cardiovascular Events and Deaths in US Adults: An Analysis of National Data," *JAMA Cardiology* 3, no. 7 (2018): 572–581.

28. S. J. Pocock and G. W. Stone, "The Primary Outcome Is Positive—Is That Good Enough?" *NEJM* 375 (2016): 971–979.

29. R. M. Kaplan, A. M. Navarro, F. G. Castro, et al., "Increased Use of Mammography among Hispanic Women: Baseline Results from the NCI Cooperative Group on Cancer Prevention in Hispanic Communities," *American Journal of Preventive Medicine* 12 (1996): 467–471.

30. A. M. Navarro and R. M. Kaplan, "Mammography Screening: Prospects and Opportunity Costs," *Women's Health* 2 (1996): 209–233.

31. M. Baum, "'Catch It Early, Save a Life and Save a Breast': This Misleading Mantra of Mammography," *Journal of the Royal Society of Medicine* 108 (2015): 338–339; N. Biller-Andorno and P. Juni, "Abolishing Mammography Screening Programs? A View from the Swiss Medical Board," *NEJM* 370 (2014): 1965–1967; A. Bleyer and H. G. Welch, "Effect of Three Decades of Screening Mammography on Breast-Cancer Incidence," *NEJM* 367 (2012): 1998–2005; A. Bleyer and H. G. Welch, response to letters to the editor, "Correspondence: Effect of Screening Mammography on Breast Cancer Incidence," *NEJM* 368 (2013): 679; J. J. Fenton, "Is It Time to Stop Paying for Computer-Aided Mammography?" *JAMA Internal Medicine* 175 (2015): 1837–1838; P. C. Gotzsche, "Mammography Screening Is Harmful and Should Be Abandoned," *Journal of the Royal Society of Medicine* 108 (2015): 341–345; P. C. Gotzsche and K. J. Jorgensen, "Screening for Breast Cancer with Mammography," *Cochrane Database of Systematic Reviews* 6 (2013): CD001877; J. D. Keen and K. J. Jorgensen, "Four Principles to Consider before Advising Women on Screening Mammography," *Journal of Women's Health* 24, no. 11 (2015): 867–874; O. Olsen and P. C. Gotzsche, "Cochrane Review on Screening for

Breast Cancer with Mammography," *Lancet* 358 (2001): 1340–1342; H. G. Welch and H. J. Passow, "Quantifying the Benefits and Harms of Screening Mammography," *JAMA Internal Medicine* 174 (2014): 448–454.

32. H. D. Nelson, R. Fu, A. Cantor, et al., "Effectiveness of Breast Cancer Screening: Systematic Review and Meta-Analysis to Update the 2009 US Preventive Services Task Force Recommendation," *Annals of Internal Medicine* 164 (2016): 244–255; D. Fitzpatrick-Lewis, N. Hodgson, D. Ciliska, et al., *Breast Cancer Screening*, Canadian Task Force on Preventive Health Care, October 7, 2011, https:// canadiantaskforce.ca/wp-content/uploads/2011/11/2011-breast-cancer-systematic -review-en.pdf; P. C. Gotzsche and K. J. Jorgensen, "Screening for Breast Cancer with Mammography," *Cochrane Database of Systematic Reviews* 6 (2013): CD001877; J. S. Mandelblatt, N. K. Stout, C. B. Schechter, et al., "Collaborative Modeling of the Benefits and Harms Associated with Different US Breast Cancer Screening Strategies," *Annals of Internal Medicine* 164, no. 4 (2016): 215–225; H. D. Nelson, K. Tyne, A. Naik, et al., "Screening for Breast Cancer: An Update for the US Preventive Services Task Force," *Annals of Internal Medicine* 151 (2009): 727–737.

33. A. B. Miller, C. J. Baines, T. To, and C. Wall, "Canadian National Breast Screening Study: 1. Breast Cancer Detection and Death Rates among Women Aged 40 to 49 Years," *Canadian Medical Association Journal* 147(1992): 1459–1476.

34. V. L. Irvin and R. M. Kaplan, "Screening Mammography and Breast Cancer Mortality: Meta-Analysis of Quasi-Experimental Studies," *PlOS One* 9 (2014): e98105.

35. A. Bleyer, C. Baines, and A. B. Miller, "Impact of Screening Mammography on Breast Cancer Mortality," *International Journal of Cancer* 138, no. 8 (2016): 2003–2012.

36. N. Biller-Andorno and P. Juni, "Abolishing Mammography Screening Programs? A View from the Swiss Medical Board," *NEJM* 370 (2014): 1965–1967.

37. A. Barratt, K. J. Jørgensen, and P. Autier, "Reform of the National Screening Mammography Program in France," *JAMA Internal Medicine* 178, no. 2 (2018): 177–178.

38. H. G. Welch and H. J. Passow, "Quantifying the Benefits and Harms of Screening Mammography," *JAMA Internal Medicine* 174 (2014): 448–454.

39. E. R. Myers, P. Moorman, J. M. Gierisch, et al., "Benefits and Harms of Breast Cancer Screening: A Systematic Review," *JAMA* 314 (2015): 1615–1634.

40. K. Staat and M. Segatore, "The Phenomenon of Chemo Brain," *Clinical Journal of Oncology Nursing* 9 (2005): 713–721.

41. S. C. Darby, M. Ewertz, P. McGale, et al., "Risk of Ischemic Heart Disease in Women after Radiotherapy for Breast Cancer," *NEJM* 368 (2013): 987–998.

42. L. M. Schwartz, S. Woloshin, F. J. Fowler Jr., and H. G. Welch, "Enthusiasm for Cancer Screening in the United States," *JAMA* 291 (2004): 71–78.

43. R. A. Aronowitz, "Do Not Delay: Breast Cancer and Time, 1900–1970," *Milbank Quarterly* 79, no. 3 (2001): 355–386.

44. H. G. Welch and H. J. Passow, "Quantifying the Benefits and Harms of Screening Mammography," *JAMA Internal Medicine* 174 (2014): 448–454.

45. W. C. Black and H. G. Welch, "Screening for Disease," *American Journal of Roentgenology* 168 (1997): 3–11.

46. T. A. Manolio, G. L. Burke, D. H. O'Leary, et al., "Relationships of Cerebral MRI Findings to Ultrasonographic Carotid Atherosclerosis in Older Adults: The Cardiovascular Health Study," *Arteriosclerosis, Thrombosis, and Vascular Biology* 19, no. 2 (1999): 356–365.

47. P. M. Marcus, E. J. Bergstralh, R. M. Fagerstrom, et al., "Lung Cancer Mortality in the Mayo Lung Project: Impact of Extended Follow-Up," *Journal of the National Cancer Instititue* 92 (2000): 1308–1316; N. Saquib, J. Saquib, and J. P. Ioannidis, "Does Screening for Disease Save Lives in Asymptomatic Adults? Systematic Review of Meta-Analyses and Randomized Trials," *International Journal of Epidemiology* 44 (2015): 264–277.

48. W. C. Black and H. G. Welch, "Screening for Disease," *American Journal of Roentgenology* 168 (1997): 3–11.

49. R. M. Kaplan, *Diseases, Diagnoses, and Dollars* (New York: Springer, 2009).

50. J. V. Selby, A. C. Beal, and L. Frank, "The Patient-Centered Outcomes Research Institute (PCORI) National Priorities for Research and Initial Research Agenda," *JAMA* 307 (2012): 1583–1584.

51. J. M. Pascoe, D. L. Wood, J. H. Duffee, and A. Kuo, "Mediators and Adverse Effects of Child Poverty in the United States," *Pediatrics* 137, no. 4 (2016): e20160340.

4. Making Health Care Safe and Effective

1. A. P. Shapiro, "Illness and Death in American Presidents," in *Behavioral Aspects of Cardiovascular Disease,* ed. A. P. Shapiro and A. Baum (New York: Psychology Press, 2014), 327–338.

2. H. G. Bruenn, "Clinical Notes on the Illness and Death of President Franklin D. Roosevelt," *Annals of Internal Medicine* 72, no.4 (1970): 579–591.

3. J. T. James, "Deaths from Preventable Adverse Events Originating in Hospitals," *BMJ Quality and Safety* 26, no. 8 (2017): 692–693; K. P. Marsack and L. H. Hollier Jr., "Review of 'Medical Error—The Third Leading Cause of Death in the US,' by M. A. Makary and M. Daniel in *BMJ* 353: i2139, 2016," *Journal of Craniofacial Surgery* 28, no. 5 (2017): 1390.

4. L. L. Leape, T. A. Brennan, N. Laird, et al., "The Nature of Adverse Events in Hospitalized Patients: Results of the Harvard Medical Practice Study II," *NEJM* 324 (1991): 377–384.

5. L. T. Kohn, J. M. Corrigan, and M. S. Donaldson, eds., *To Err Is Human: Building a Safer Health System* (Washington, DC: National Academies Press, 2000).

6. C. J. McDonald, M. Weiner, and S. L. Hui, "Deaths Due to Medical Errors Are Exaggerated in Institute of Medicine Report," *JAMA* 284 (2000): 93–95; L. L. Leape, "Institute of Medicine Medical Error Figures Are Not Exaggerated," *JAMA* 284 (2000): 95–97.

7. J. T. James, "A New, Evidence-Based Estimate of Patient Harms Associated with Hospital Care," *Journal of Patient Safety* 9 (2013): 122–128.

8. E. P. Balogh, B. T. Miller, and J. R. Ball, eds., *Improving Diagnosis in Health Care* (Washington, DC: National Academies Press, 2015).

9. B. Nelson, "The Right Prescriptions for Reducing Diagnostic Errors? Institute of Medicine Report Issues Wakeup Call on Errors, but Questions Remain Concerning Key Recommendations," *Cancer Cytopathology* 124 (2016): 77–78.

10. H. Singh and L. Zwaan, "Annals for Hospitalists Inpatient Notes-Reducing Diagnostic Error—A New Horizon of Opportunities for Hospital MedicineInpatient Notes: Reducing Diagnostic Error," *Annals of Internal Medicine* 165, no. 8 (2016): HO2–HO4.

11. G. Neta, R. E. Glasgow, C. R. Carpenter, et al., "A Framework for Enhancing the Value of Research for Dissemination and Implementation," *American Journal of Public Health* 105 (2015): 49–57.

12. H. G. Welch, D. H. Gorski, and P. C. Albertsen, "Trends in Metastatic Breast and Prostate Cancer—Lessons in Cancer Dynamics," *NEJM* 373 (2015): 1685–1687.

13. T. Montini and I. D. Graham, "'Entrenched Practices and Other Biases': Unpacking the Historical, Economic, Professional, and Social Resistance to De-implementation," *Implementation Science* 10 (2015): 24.

14. S. Mukherjee, *The Emperor of All Maladies: A Biography of Cancer* (New York: Scribner, 2011).

15. R. M. Kaplan and F. Porzsolt, "The Natural History of Breast Cancer," *Archives of Internal Medicine* 168 (2008): 2302–2303.

16. H. G. Welch, D. H. Gorski, and P. C. Albertsen, "Trends in Metastatic Breast and Prostate Cancer—Lessons in Cancer Dynamics," *NEJM* 373 (2015): 1685–1687.

17. B. Fisher, C. Redmond, R. Poisson, et al., "Eight-Year Results of a Randomized Clinical Trial Comparing Total Mastectomy and Lumpectomy with or without Irradiation in the Treatment of Breast Cancer," *NEJM* 320 (1989): 822–828.

18. B. Fisher, S. Anderson, J. Bryant, et al., "Twenty-Year Follow-Up of a Randomized Trial Comparing Total Mastectomy, Lumpectomy, and Lumpectomy Plus Irradiation for the Treatment of Invasive Breast Cancer," *NEJM* 347 (2002): 1233–1241.

19. Agency of Healthcare Research and Quality, "National Patient Safety Efforts Save 125,000 Lives and Nearly $28 Billion in Costs," press release, December 12, 2016, https://www.ahrq.gov/news/newsroom/press-releases/national-patient-safety-efforts-save-lives.html.

20. P. Pronovost, D. Needham, S. Berenholtz, et al., "An Intervention to Decrease Catheter-Related Bloodstream Infections in the ICU," *NEJM* 355 (2006): 2725–2732.

21. A. Gawande, *The Checklist Manifesto* (New York: Metropolitan Books, 2010).

22. P. Pronovost, D. Needham, S. Berenholtz, et al., "An Intervention to Decrease Catheter-Related Bloodstream Infections in the ICU," *NEJM* 355 (2006): 2725–2732.

23. D. J. Anderson, K. Podgorny, S. I. Berríos-Torres, et al., "Strategies to Prevent Surgical Site Infections in Acute Care Hospitals: 2014 Update," *Infection Control and Hospital Epidemiology* 35 (2014): S66-S88.

24. C. P. Cannon, C. M. Gibson, C. T. Lambrew, et al., "Relationship of Symptom-Onset-to-Balloon Time and Door-to-Balloon Time with Mortality in Patients Undergoing Angioplasty for Acute Myocardial Infarction," *JAMA* 238 (2000): 2941–2947.

25. M. B. Yudi, G. Hamilton, O. Farouque, et al., "Trends and Impact of Door-to-Balloon Time on Clinical Outcomes in Patients Aged <75, 75 to 84,

and ≥ 85 Years with ST-Elevation Myocardial Infarction," *American Journal of Cardiology* 120 (2017): 1245–1253.

26. G. C. Fonarow, X. Zhao, E. E. Smith, et al., "Door-to-Needle Times for Tissue Plasminogen Activator Administration and Clinical Outcomes in Acute Ischemic Stroke before and after a Quality Improvement Initiative," *JAMA* 311 (2014): 1632–1640.

27. W. V. Crandall, P. A. Margolis, M. D. Kappelman, et al., "Improved Outcomes in a Quality Improvement Collaborative for Pediatric Inflammatory Bowel Disease," *Pediatrics* 129 (2012): e1030–e1041.

28. R. D. Fletcher, R. L. Amdur, R. Kheirbek, et al., "Blood Pressure Control That Reduces Mortality and Cardiovascular Events from 2000 to 2014 for Patients in the Veterans Administration Healthcare System," *Circulation* 134, suppl. 1 (2016): A17842.

29. Blood Pressure Lowering Treatment Trialists' Collaboration, "Effects of Different Blood-Pressure-Lowering Regimens on Major Cardiovascular Events: Results of Prospectively-Designed Overviews of Randomised Trials," *Lancet* 362 (2003): 1527–1535.

30. W. C. Cushman, P. K. Whelton, L. J. Fine, et al., "SPRINT Trial Results," *Hypertension* 67 (2016): 263–265.

31. W. B. Kannel, T. R. Dawber, A. Kagan, et al., "Factors of Risk in the Development of Coronary Heart Disease—Six-Year Follow-Up Experience: The Framingham Study," *Annals of Internal Medicine* 55 (1961): 33–50.

32. I. Hajjar and T. A. Kotchen, "Trends in Prevalence, Awareness, Treatment, and Control of Hypertension in the United States, 1988–2000," *JAMA* 290 (2003): 199–206.

33. K. L. Ong, B. M. Cheung, Y. B. Man, et al., "Prevalence, Awareness, Treatment, and Control of Hypertension Among United States Adults 1999–2004," *Hypertension* 49 (2007): 69–75.

34. M. G. Jaffe, G. A. Lee, J. D. Young, S. Sidney, and A. S. Go, "Improved Blood Pressure Control Associated with a Large-Scale Hypertension Program," *JAMA* 310, no. 7 (2013): 699–705.

35. R. M. Kaplan, Z. Fang, and G. Morgan, "Providers' Advice Concerning Smoking Cessation: Evidence from the Medical Expenditures Panel Survey," *Preventive Medicine* 91 (2016): 32–36.

36. B. D. Fulton, S. L. Ivey, H. P. Rodriguez, and S. M. Shortell, "Countywide Physician Organization Learning Collaborative and Changes in Hospitalization Rates," *American Journal of Managed Care* 23 (2017): 596–603.

5. Social Determinants of Health

1. T. C. Timmreck, *An Introduction to Epidemiology* (Boston: Jones and Bartlett, 1994); J. Snow, W. H. Frost, and B. W. Richardson, *Snow on Cholera, Being a Reprint of Two Papers by John Snow* (New York: Commonwealth Fund, 1936).

2. R. M. Kaplan, J. F. Sallis, and T. L. Patterson, *Health and Human Behavior* (New York: McGraw-Hill, 1993).

3. D. L. Hoyert and J. Xu, "Deaths: Preliminary Data for 2011," *National Vital Statistics Report* 61, no. 6 (2012): 1–51.

4. E. Bradley and L. Taylor, *The American Health Care Paradox: Why Spending More Is Getting Us Less* (New York: PublicAffairs, 2013).

5. R. Tjian, "Supporting Biomedical Research: Meeting Challenges and Opportunities at HHMI," *JAMA* 313 (2015): 133–134.

6. Strategic Review of Health Inequalities in England Post-2010 (M. Marmot, J. Allen, P. Goldblatt, et al.), "Fair Society, Healthy Lives (The Marmot Report)," Institute of Health Equity, London, February 2010, http://www.instituteofhealthequity.org/resources-reports/fair-society-healthy-lives-the-marmot-review/fair-society-healthy-lives-full-report-pdf.pdf.

7. P. A. Braveman, S. Kumanyika, J. Fielding, et al., "Health Disparities and Health Equity: The Issue Is Justice," *American Journal of Public Health* 101, suppl. 1 (2011): S149–S155.

8. C. J. Murray, S. C. Kulkarni, C. Michaud, et al., "Eight Americas: Investigating Mortality Disparities across Races, Counties, and Race-Counties in the United States," *PLOS Medicine* 3 (2006): e260.

9. Murray, Kulkarni, Michaud, et al., "Eight Americas."

10. R. Chetty, M. Stepner, S. Abraham, et al., "The Association between Income and Life Expectancy in the United States, 2001–2014," *JAMA* 315 (2016): 1750–1766.

11. R. G. Wilkinson and K. E. Pickett, *The Spirit Level: Why Equality Is Better for Everyone* (London: Allen Lane, 2009).

12. K. E. Pickett and R. G. Wilkinson, "Income Inequality and Health: A Causal Review," *Social Science and Medicine* 128 (2015): 316–326.

13. D. Pillas, M. Marmot, K. Naicker, et al., "Social Inequalities in Early Childhood Health and Development: A European-Wide Systematic Review," *Pediatric Research* 76 (2014): 418–424.

14. Council on Community Pediatrics, "Poverty and Child Health in the United States," *Pediatrics* 137 (2016): 1–28.

15. K. Seefeldt and J. D. Graham, *America's Poor and the Great Recession* (Bloomington: Indiana University Press, 2013).

16. C. DeNavas-Walt and B. D. Proctor, "Income and Poverty in the United States: 2013," Current Population Reports, P60-249, United States Census Bureau, Washington, DC, September 2014, https://www.census.gov/content/dam/Census/library/publications/2014/demo/p60-249.pdf.

17. C. DeNavas-Walt and B. D. Proctor, "Income and Poverty in the United States: 2014," Current Population Reports, P60-252, United States Census Bureau, Washington, DC, September 2015, https://www.census.gov/content/dam/Census/library/publications/2015/demo/p60-252.pdf.

18. L. Fox, I. Garfinkel, N. Kaushal, et al., "Waging War on Poverty: Historical Trends in Poverty Using the Supplemental Poverty Measure," *Journal of Policy Analysis and Management* 34, no. 3 (2015): 567–592.

19. M. R. Cullen, C. Cummins, and V. R. Fuchs, "Geographic and Racial Variation in Premature Mortality in the U.S.: Analyzing the Disparities," *PLOS One* 7, no. 4 (2012): e32930.

20. D. R. Williams, N. Priest, and N. B. Anderson, "Understanding Associations among Race, Socioeconomic Status, and Health: Patterns and Prospects," *Health Psychology* 35, no. 4 (2016): 407–411.

21. C. D. Gillespie, C. Wigington, Y. Hong, "Coronary Heart Disease and Stroke Deaths—United States, 2009," *Morbidity and Mortality Weekly Report* 62, no. 3 (2013): 157–160.

22. D. R. Williams, N. Priest, and N. B. Anderson, "Understanding Associations among Race, Socioeconomic Status, and Health: Patterns and Prospects," *Health Psychology* 35, no. 4 (2016): 407–411.

23. Williams, Priest, and Anderson, "Understanding Associations."

24. A. Smedley and B. D. Smedley, "Race as Biology Is Fiction, Racism as a Social Problem Is Real: Anthropological and Historical Perspectives on the Social Construction of Race," *American Psychologist* 60, no. 1 (2005): 16–26.

25. O. W. Brawley and H. P. Freeman, "Race and Outcomes: Is This the End of the Beginning for Minority Health Research?" *Journal of the National Cancer Institute* 91, no. 22 (1999): 1908–1909.

26. H. P. Freeman and R. Payne, "Racial Injustice in Health Care," *NEJM* 342, no. 14 (2000): 1045–1047; M. Ellis, *Race and Medicine in Nineteenth and Early Twentieth-Century America* (Oxford: Oxford University Press, 2008).

27. J. M. Metzl and D. E. Roberts, "Structural Competency Meets Structural Racism: Race, Politics, and the Structure of Medical Knowledge," *Virtual Mentor* 16, no. 9 (2014): 674–690.

28. G. Markowitz and D. Rosner, *Deceit and Denial: The Deadly Politics of Industrial Pollution,* (Berkeley: University of California Press, 2013).

29. M. Hanna-Attisha, J. LaChance, R. C. Sadler, and A. Champney Schnepp, "Elevated Blood Lead Levels in Children Associated with the Flint Drinking Water Crisis: A Spatial Analysis of Risk and Public Health Response," *American Journal of Public Health* 106, no. 2 (2016): 283–290.

30. S. Zahran, S. P. McElmurry, P. E. Kilgore, et al., "Assessment of the Legionnaires' Disease Outbreak in Flint, Michigan," *PNAS* 115, no. 8 (2018): E1730–E1739.

31. P. Egan, "Flint Mayor: Cost of Lead Fix Could Hit $1.5 Billion," *Detroit Free Press,* January 7, 2016, http://www.freep.com/story/news/local/michigan/2016/01/07/governor-meet-morning-flint-mayor/78402190/.

32. S. B. Hong, M. H. Im, J. W. Kim, et al., "Environmental Lead Exposure and Attention Deficit/Hyperactivity Disorder Symptom Domains in a Community Sample of South Korean School-Age Children," *Environmental Health Perspectives* 123, no. 3 (2015): 271–276.

33. K. F. Ferraro, M. H. Schafer, and L. R. Wilkinson, "Childhood Disadvantage and Health Problems in Middle and Later Life," *American Sociological Review* 81, no. 1 (2016): 107–133.

34. R. J. Sampson and A. S. Winter, "The Racial Ecology of Lead Poisoning: Toxic Inequality in Chicago Neighborhoods, 1995–2013," *Du Bois Review: Social Science Research on Race* 13 (2016): 261–283.

35. J. B. Dowd, T. Palermo, L. Chyu, E. Adam, and T. W. McDade, "Race/Ethnic and Socioeconomic Differences in Stress and Immune Function in the National Longitudinal Study of Adolescent Health," *Social Science and Medicine* 115 (2014): 49–55.

36. R. T. Carter, M. Y. Llau, V. Johnson, and K. Kirkinis, "Racial Discrimination and Health Outcomes among Racial/Ethnic Minorities: A Meta-Analytic Review," *Journal of Multicultural Counseling and Development* 45, no. 4 (2017): 232–259.

37. L. F. Berkman and L. O Kawachi, eds. *Social Epidemiology* (Oxford: Oxford University Press, 2000); S. C. Maty, J. W. Lynch, T. E. Raghunathan, et al., "Childhood Socioeconomic Position, Gender, Adult Body Mass Index, and Incidence of Type 2 Diabetes Mellitus over 34 Years in the Alameda County Study," *American Journal of Public Health* 98, no. 8 (2008): 1486–1494; G. Turrell, J. W. Lynch, C. Leite, et al., "Socioeconomic Disadvantage in Childhood and across the Life Course and All-Cause Mortality and Physical Function in Adulthood: Evidence from the Alameda County Study," *Journal of Epidemiology and Community Health* 61, no. 8 (2007): 723–730; I. H. Yen and G. A. Kaplan, "Neighborhood Social Environment and Risk of Death: Multilevel Evidence from the Alameda County Study," *American Journal of Epidemiology* 149 (1999): 898–907.

38. Yen and Kaplan, "Neighborhood Social Environment."

39. Maty, Lynch, Raghunathan, et al., "Childhood Socioeconomic Position"; Turrell, Lynch, Leite, et al., "Socioeconomic Disadvantage in Childhood."

40. T. E. Seeman, G. A. Kaplan, L. Knudsen, et al., "Social Network Ties and Mortality among the Elderly in the Alameda County Study," *American Journal of Epidemiology* 126 (1987): 714–723; V. Johnson-Lawrence, S. Galea, and G. A. Kaplan, "Cumulative Socioeconomic Disadvantage and Cardiovascular Disease Mortality in the Alameda County Study 1965 to 2000," *Annals of Epidemiology* 25 (2015): 65–70.

41. A. Steptoe, A. Shankar, P. Demakakos, and J. Wardle, "Social Isolation, Loneliness, and All-Cause Mortality in Older Men and Women," *PNAS* 110 (2013): 5797–5801.

42. R. M. Kaplan and R. G. Kronick, "Marital Status and Longevity in the United States Population," *Journal of Epidemiology and Community Health* 60 (2006): 760–765.

43. S. Stringhini, L. Berkman, A. Dugravot, et al., "Socioeconomic Status, Structural and Functional Measures of Social Support, and Mortality: The British Whitehall II Cohort Study, 1985–2009," *American Journal of Epidemiology* 175 (2012): 1275–1283.

44. L. F. Berkman, "Assessing the Physical Health Effects of Social Networks and Social Support," *Annual Review of Public Health* 5 (1984): 413–432.

45. J. Holt-Lunstad, T. B. Smith, M. Baker, et al., "Loneliness and Social Isolation as Risk Factors for Mortality," *Perspectives on Psychological Science* 10, no. 2 (2015): 227–237.

46. J. T. Cacioppo, S. Cacioppo, S. W. Cole, et al., "Loneliness across Phylogeny and a Call for Comparative Studies and Animal Models," *Perspectives on Psychological Science* 10, no. 2 (2015): 202–212.

47. M. L. Laudenslager, T. L. Simoneau, S. Philips, et al., "A Randomized Controlled Pilot Study of Inflammatory Gene Expression in Response to a

Stress Management Intervention for Stem Cell Transplant Caregivers," *Journal of Behavioral Medicine* 39, no. 2 (2016): 346–354.

48. J. K. Montez, R. A. Hummer, and M. D. Hayward, "Educational Attainment and Adult Mortality in the United States: A Systematic Analysis of Functional Form," *Demography* 49, no. 1 (2012): 315–336.

49. J. K. Montez, R. A. Hummer, M. D. Hayward, et al., "Trends in the Educational Gradient of U.S. Adult Mortality from 1986 through 2006 by Race, Gender, and Age Group," *Research on Aging* 33, no. 2 (2011): 145–171.

50. S. J. Olshansky, T. Antonucci, L. Berkman, et al., "Differences in Life Expectancy due to Race and Educational Differences Are Widening, and Many May Not Catch Up," *Health Affairs* 31, no. 8 (2012): 1803–1813.

51. R. G. Rogers, B. G. Everett, A. Zajacova, and R. A. Hummer, "Educational Degrees and Adult Mortality Risk in the United States," *Biodemography and Social Biology* 56, no. 1 (2010): 80–99; J. K. Montez, M. D. Hayward, D. C. Brown, and R. Hummer, "Why Is the Educational Gradient of Mortality Steeper for Men?" *Journals of Gerontology B: Psychological Sciences and Social Sciences* 64B, no. 5 (2009): 625–634.

52. A. Zajacova, R. A. Hummer, and R. G. Rogers, "Education and Health among U.S. Working-Age Adults: A Detailed Portrait across the Full Educational Attainment Spectrum," *Biodemography and Social Biology* 58, no. 1 (2012): 40–61.

53. R. M. Kaplan, V. J. Howard, M. M. Safford, and G. Howard, "Educational Attainment and Longevity: Results from the REGARDS U.S. National Cohort Study of Blacks and Whites," *Annals of Epidemiology* 25, no. 5 (2015): 323–328.

54. J. Ma, J. Xu, R. N. Anderson, and A. Jemal, "Widening Educational Disparities in Premature Death Rates in Twenty Six States in the United States, 1993–2007," *PlOS One* 7 (2012): e41560.

55. P. C. Gotzsche and K. J. Jorgensen, "Screening for Breast Cancer with Mammography," *Cochrane Database of Systematic Reviews,* no. 1 (2011): CD001877.

56. R. Clarke, J. Emberson, A. Fletcher, et al., "Life Expectancy in Relation to Cardiovascular Risk Factors: 38 Year Follow-Up of 19,000 Men in the Whitehall Study," *BMJ* 339, no. 7725 (2009): b3513.

57. J. K. Montez and M. D. Hayward, "Cumulative Childhood Adversity, Educational Attainment, and Active Life Expectancy among U.S. Adults," *Demography* 51, no. 2 (2014): 413–435.

58. S. Galea, M. Tracy, J. Hoggatt, et al., "Estimated Deaths Attributable to Social Factors in the United States," *American Journal of Public Health* 101, no. 8 (2011): 1456–1465.

59. J. Mirowsky, *Education, Social Status, and Health* (New York: Routledge, 2017).

60. D. M. Cutler and A. Lleras-Muney, "Understanding Differences in Health Behaviors by Education," *Journal of Health Economics* 29, no. 1 (2010): 1–28.

61. N. Adler, M. S. Pantell, A. O'Donovan, et al., "Educational Attainment and Late Life Telomere Length in the Health, Aging and Body Composition Study," *Brain Behavior and Immunity* 27 (2013): 15–21.

62. D. Clark, and H. Royer, "The Effect of Education on Adult Mortality and Health: Evidence from Britain," *American Economic Review* 103, no. 6 (2013): 2087–2120.

63. Institute of Medicine, *Capturing Social and Behavioral Domains and Measures in Electronic Health Records: Phase 2* (Washington DC: National Academies Press, 2014), https://www.ncbi.nlm.nih.gov/books/NBK268995/pdf/Bookshelf _NBK268995.pdf.

64. A. L. Plough, "Building a Culture of Health: Challenges for the Public Health Workforce," *American Journal of Preventive Medicine* 47, no. 5 (2014): S388–S390.

65. J. O'Donnell, "Feds to Study Health Benefits of Screening and Linking to Social Services," *USA Today,* February 3, 2016.

66. E. H. Bradley, M. Canavan, E. Rogan, et al., "Variation in Health Outcomes: The Role of Spending on Social Services, Public Health, and Health Care, 2000–09," *Health Affairs* 35 (2016): 760–768.

6. The Act of Well-Being

1. N. J. Stone, J. G Robinson, A. H. Lichtenstein, et al., "Treatment of Blood Cholesterol to Reduce Atherosclerotic Cardiovascular Disease Risk in Adults: Synopsis of the 2013 American College of Cardiology / American Heart Association Cholesterol Guideline," *Annals of Internal Medicine* 160 (2014): 339–343.

2. S. J. Olshansky, D. J. Passaro, R. C. Hershow, et al., "A Potential Decline in Life Expectancy in the United States in the 21st Century," *NEJM* 352 (2005): 1138–1145.

3. "Overdose Death Rates," National Institute of Drug Abuse, last modified September 2017, https://www.drugabuse.gov/related-topics/trends-statistics /overdose-death-rates.

4. T. Gomes, M. Tadrous, M. M. Mamdani, J. M. Paterson, and D. N. Juurlink, "The Burden of Opioid-Related Mortality in the United States," *JAMA Network Open* 1, no. 2 (2018): e180217–e180217.

5. G. Kolata and S. Cohen, "Drug Overdoses Propel Rise in Mortality Rates of Young Whites," *New York Times,* January 17, 2016.

6. R. J. Gatchel, D. D. McGeary, C. A. McGeary, and B. Lippe, "Interdisciplinary Chronic Pain Management: Past, Present, and Future," *American Psychologist* 69 (2014): 119–130.

7. US Department of Health and Human Services, *The Health Consequences of Smoking—50 Years of Progress: A Report of the Surgeon General* (Atlanta: USDHHS, Centers for Disease Control and Prevention, National Center for Chronic Disease Prevention and Health Promotion, Office on Smoking and Health, 2014), https://www.ncbi.nlm.nih.gov/books/NBK179276/.

8. US Department of Health and Human Services, *The Health Consequences of Smoking,* https://www.ncbi.nlm.nih.gov/books/NBK179276/.

9. US Department of Health and Human Services, *The Health Consequences of Smoking,* https://www.ncbi.nlm.nih.gov/books/NBK179276/.

10. US Department of Health and Human Services, *The Health Consequences of Smoking*, https://www.ncbi.nlm.nih.gov/books/NBK179276/.

11. R. N. Proctor, *Golden Holocaust: Origins of the Cigarette Catastrophe and the Case for Abolition* (Berkeley: University of California Press, 2011); R. N. Proctor, "Why Ban the Sale of Cigarettes? The Case for Abolition," *Tobacco Control* 22, suppl. 1 (2013): i27–i30.

12. D. B. Abrams, A. M. Glasser, A. C. Villanti, and R. Niaura, "Cigarettes: The Rise and Decline but Not Demise of the Greatest Behavioral Health Disaster of the 20th Century," in *Population Health: Behavioral and Social Science Insights,* ed. R. M. Kaplan, M. L. Spittel, and D. H. David, AHRQ Pub. No. 15-0002 (Rockville, MD: Agency for Healthcare Research and Quality and Office of Behavioral and Social Sciences Research, National Institutes of Health, 2015), 143–168.

13. P. Jha and R. Peto, "Global Effects of Smoking, of Quitting, and of Taxing Tobacco," *NEJM* 370 (2014): 60–68.

14. N. K. Cobb and D. B. Abrams, "The FDA, E-Cigarettes, and the Demise of Combusted Tobacco," *NEJM* 371 (2014): 1469–1471.

15. Jha and Peto, "Global Effects of Smoking."

16. J. F. Sallis and J. A. Carlson, "Physical Activity: Numerous Benefits and Effective Interventions," in *Population Health: Behavioral and Social Science Insights,* ed. R. M. Kaplan, M. L. Spittel, and D. H. David, AHRQ Pub. No. 15-0002 (Rockville, MD: Agency for Healthcare Research and Quality and Office of Behavioral and Social Sciences Research, National Institutes of Health, 2015), 169–184.

17. I. M. Lee, E. J. Shiroma, F. Lobelo, et al., "Effect of Physical Inactivity on Major Non-Communicable Diseases Worldwide: An Analysis of Burden of Disease and Life Expectancy," *Lancet* 380 (2012): 219–229.

18. D. A. Glei, F. Mesle, Jacques Vallin, et al., "Diverging Trends in Life Expectancy at Age 50: A Look at Causes of Death," in *International Differences in Mortality at Older Ages: Dimensions and Sources,* ed. E. M. Crimmins, S. H. Preston, and B. Cohen (Washington, DC: National Academies Press, 2010), 385–408.

19. G. O'Donovan, I. M. Lee, M. Hamer, and E. Stamatakis, "Association of 'Weekend Warrior' and Other Leisure Time Physical Activity Patterns with Risks for All-Cause, Cardiovascular Disease, and Cancer Mortality," *JAMA Internal Medicine* 177 (2017): 335–342.

20. D. C. Lee, A. G. Brellenthin, P. D. Thompson, et al., "Running as a Key Lifestyle Medicine for Longevity," *Progress in Cardiovascular Diseases* 60, no. 1 (2017): 45–55.

21. P. Heyn, B. C. Abreu, and K. J. Ottenbacher, "The Effects of Exercise Training on Elderly Persons with Cognitive Impairment and Dementia: A Meta-Analysis," *Archives of Physical Medicine and Rehabilitation* 85 (2004): 1694–1704.

22. G. T. Keusch, "The History of Nutrition: Malnutrition, Infection and Immunity," *Journal of Nutrition* 133 (2003): 336S–340S.

23. "Adult Obesity Facts," Overweight and Obesity, Centers for Disease Control and Prevention, 2014, https://www.cdc.gov/obesity/data/adult.html.

24. C. L. Ogden, M. D. Carroll, B. K. Kit, and K. M. Flegal, "Prevalence of Obesity and Trends in Body Mass Index among US Children and Adolescents, 1999–2010," *JAMA* 307 (2012): 483–490; D. B. Allison, K. R. Fontaine, J. E. Manson, et al., "Annual Deaths Attributable to Obesity in the United States," *JAMA* 282 (1999): 1530–1538.

25. E. J. Groessl, R. M. Kaplan, E. Barrett-Connor, and T. G. Ganiats, "Body Mass Index and Quality of Well-Being in a Community of Older Adults," *American Journal of Preventive Medicine* 26 (2004): 126–129; E. A. Finkelstein, I. C. Fiebelkorn, and G. Wang, "National Medical Spending Attributable to Overweight and Obesity: How Much, and Who's Paying?" *Health Affairs* (2003), suppl. web exclusive, W3-219-26; E. A. Finkelstein, C. J. Ruhm, and K. M. Kosa, "Economic Causes and Consequences of Obesity," *Annual Review of Public Health* 26 (2005): 239–257; E. A. Finkelstein, J. G. Trogdon, J. W. Cohen, and W. Dietz, "Annual Medical Spending Attributable to Obesity: Payer- and Service-Specific Estimates," *Health Affairs* 28 (2009): w822–w831.

26. D. D. Kim and A. Basu, "Estimating the Medical Care Costs of Obesity in the United States: Systematic Review, Meta-Analysis, and Empirical Analysis," *Value in Health* 19 (2016): 602–613.

27. K. M. Flegal, M. D. Carroll, B. K. Kit, and C. L. Ogden, "Prevalence of Obesity and Trends in the Distribution of Body Mass Index among US Adults, 1999–2010," *JAMA* 307 (2012): 491–497; C. M. Hales, M. D. Carroll, C. D. Fryar, and C. L. Ogden, "Prevalence of Obesity among Adults and Youth: United States, 2015–2016," NCHS Data Brief no. 288, October 2017, National Center for Health Statistics, Centers for Disease Control, https://www.cdc.gov/nchs/data/databriefs/db288.pdf.

28. C. L. Ogden, M. D. Carroll, B. K. Kit, and K. M. Flegal, "Prevalence of Obesity and Trends in Body Mass Index among US Children and Adolescents, 1999–2010," *JAMA* 307 (2012): 483–490.

29. A. S. Singh, C. Mulder, J. W. Twisk, et al., "Tracking of Childhood Overweight into Adulthood: A Systematic Review of the Literature," *Obesity Reviews* 9, no. 5 (2008): 474–488; D. Mozaffarian, E. J. Benjamin, A. S. Go, et al., "Heart Disease and Stroke Statistics—2015 Update: A Report from the American Heart Association," *Circulation* 131, no. 4 (2015): e29–e322; R. D. Feinman, W. K. Pogozelski, A. Astrup, et al., "Dietary Carbohydrate Restriction as the First Approach in Diabetes Management: Critical Review and Evidence Base," *Nutrition* 31, no. 1 (2015): 1–13; T. Norat, C. Scoccianti, M. C. Boutron-Ruault, et al., "European Code against Cancer 4th Edition: Diet and Cancer," *Cancer Epidemiology* 39 (2015): S56–S66; L. Schwingshackl and G. Hoffmann, "Mediterranean Dietary Pattern, Inflammation and Endothelial Function: A Systematic Review and Meta-analysis of Intervention Trials," *Nutrition, Metabolism and Cardiovascular Diseases* 24, no. 9 (2014): 929–939.

30. J. Shen, K. A. Wilmot, N. Ghasemzadeh, et al., "Mediterranean Dietary Patterns and Cardiovascular Health," *Annual Review of Nutrition* 35 (2015): 425–449.

31. Shen, Wilmot, Ghasemzadeh, et al., "Mediterranean Dietary Patterns."

32. S. Yusuf, S. Hawken, S. Ounpuu, et al., "Effect of Potentially Modifiable Risk Factors Associated with Myocardial Infarction in 52 Countries (the

INTERHEART Study): Case-Control Study," *Lancet* 364, no. 9438 (2004): 937–952.

33. M. L. Bertoia, E. W. Triche, D. S. Michaud, et al., "Mediterranean and Dietary Approaches to Stop Hypertension Dietary Patterns and Risk of Sudden Cardiac Death in Postmenopausal Women," *American Journal of Clinical Nutrition* 99, no. 2 (2014): 344–351.

34. F. Sofi, F. Cesari, R. Abbate, et al., "Adherence to Mediterranean Diet and Health Status: Meta-Analysis," *BMJ* 337, no. 7671 (2008): 673–675.

35. A. Trichopoulou, T. Costacou, C. Bamia C, and D. Trichopoulos, "Adherence to a Mediterranean Diet and Survival in a Greek Population," *NEJM* 348, no. 26 (2003): 2599–2608.

36. R. Micha, J. L. Peñalvo, F. Cudhea, et al., "Association between Dietary Factors and Mortality from Heart Disease, Stroke, and Type 2 Diabetes in the United States," *JAMA* 317, no. 9 (2017): 912–924.

37. F. F. Zhang, J. Liu, C. D. Rehm, P. Wilde, J. R. Mande, and D. Mozaffarian, "Trends and Disparities in Diet Quality Among US Adults by Supplemental Nutrition Assistance Program Participation Status," *JAMA Network Open* 1, no. 2 (2018): e180237–e180237.

38. E. B. Fisher, M. L. Fitzgibbon, R. E. Glasgow, et al. "Behavior Matters," *American Journal of Preventive Medicine* 40 (2011): e15–e30.

39. D. G. Meyers, J. S. Neuberger, J. He, "Cardiovascular Effect of Bans on Smoking in Public Places: A Systematic Review and Meta-Analysis," *Journal of the American College of Cardiology* 54, no. 14 (2009): 1249–1255.

40. K. D. Brownell and J. L. Pomeranz, "The Trans-Fat Ban—Food Regulation and Long-Term Health," *NEJM* 370 (2014): 1773–1775.

41. D. Mozaffarian, M. B. Katan, A. Ascherio, et al., "Trans Fatty Acids and Cardiovascular Disease," *NEJM* 354 (2006):1601–1613.

42. M. R. L'Abbé, S. Stender, C. Skeaff, and M. Tavella, "Approaches to Removing Trans Fats from the Food Supply in Industrialized and Developing Countries," *European Journal of Clinical Nutrition* 63 (2009): S50–S67.

43. O. Elbek, O. Kılınç, Z. A. Aytemur, et al., "Tobacco Control in Turkey," *Turkish Thoracic Journal* 16, no. 3 (2015): 141–150.

44. World Health Organization, *Global Status Report on Noncommunicable Diseases 2014* (Geneva: World Health Association, 2014), 88, http://apps.who .int/iris/bitstream/handle/10665/148114/9789241564854_en.

45. M. A. Cochero, J. Rivera-Dommarco, B. M. Popkin, and S. W. Ng., "In Mexico, Evidence of Sustained Consumer Response Two Years after Implementing a Sugar-Sweetened Beverage Tax," *Health Affairs* 36, no. 3 (2017): 564–571.

46. World Health Organization, *Global Status Report on Noncommunicable Diseases 2014* (Geneva: World Health Association, 2014), http://apps.who.int/iris /bitstream/handle/10665/148114/9789241564854_en.

47. A. S. Relman and M. Angell, "Resolved: Psychosocial Interventions Can Improve Clinical Outcomes in Organic Disease (Con)," *Psychosomatic Medicine* 64, no. 4 (2002): 558–563.

48. R. M. Kaplan and V. L. Irvin, "Likelihood of Null Effects of Large NHLBI Clinical Trials Has Increased over Time," *PLOS One* 10 (2015): e0132382.

49. V. L. Irvin and R. M. Kaplan, "Effect Sizes and Primary Outcomes in Large-Budget, Cardiovascular-Related Behavioral Randomized Controlled Trials Funded by NIH since 1980," *Annals of Behavioral Medicine* 50, no. 1 (2016): 130–146.

50. Irvin and Kaplan, "Effect Sizes and Primary Outcomes.".

51. Kaplan and Irvin, "Likelihood of Null Effects."

52. *FY 1990 Appropriation for the National Institutes of Health: Hearing Before the Subcommitte on Labor-Health and Human Services–Education, U.S. House of Representatives Committee on Appropriations*, 101st Cong. (May 1, 1989) (testimony of S. Scarr, president of the American Psychological Association).

53. R. M. Kaplan, S. Bennett-Johnson, and P. C. Kobor, "NIH Behavioral and Social Sciences Research Support: 1980–2016," *American Psychologist* 72, no. 8 (2017): 808–821.

54. B. Healy, "Health and Behavior Research 10-Year Plan," National Institutes of Health, Bethesda, MD, 1992.

55. G. C. Lee and S. Jonas, "A Proportional Funding Approach to Understanding Extramural Behavioral and Social Sciences Research and Basic Behavioral and Social Sciences Research in the NIH's Research and Basic Disease Categorization (RCDC) System," Science and Technology Policy Institute, Washington, DC, 2013.

56. R. M. Kaplan, S. B. Johnson, and P. C. Kobor, "NIH Behavioral and Social Sciences Research Support: 1980–2016," *American Psychologist* 72 (2017) 808–821.

57. R. Patterson, "Precision Medicine and Public Health: The Science of Dissemination and Implementation (PowerPoint presentation, Science of Dissemination and Implementation metting , Washington, DC, 2015).

58. R. M. Kaplan, Z. Fang, and G. Morgan, "Providers' Advice Concerning Smoking Cessation: Evidence from the Medical Expenditures Panel Survey," *Preventive Medicine* 91 (2016): 32–36.

59. Kaplan and Morgan, "Provider's Advice Concerning Smoking Cessation."

7. A Way Forward

1. S. H. Woolf and L. Y. Aron, "Failing Health of the United States: The Role of Challenging Life Conditions and the Policies behind Them," *BMJ* 360 (2018): K496.

2. D. R. Williams, N. Priest, and N. B. Anderson, "Understanding Associations among Race, Socioeconomic Status, and Health: Patterns and Prospects," *Health Psychology* 35, no. 4 (2016): 407–411.

3. C. Chanfreau-Coffinier, S. M. Teutsch, and J. E. Fielding, "Assessing the Population Impact of Published Intervention Studies," Discussion Paper, Institute of Medicine, Washington, DC, June 23, 2015, https://nam.edu/wp-content/uploads/2015/06/PopulationImpactPublishedInterventionStudies.pdf.

4. M. J. Joyner, N. Paneth, and J. P. Ioannidis, "What Happens When Underperforming Big Ideas in Research Become Entrenched?" *JAMA* 316, no. 13 (2016): 1355–1356.

5. J. L. Dieleman, E. Squires, A. L. Bui, et al., "Factors Associated with Increases in US Health Care Spending, 1996–2013," *JAMA* 318 (2017): 1668–1678.

6. V. R. Fuchs, "Major Concepts of Health Care Economics," *Annals of Internal Medicine* 162 (2015): 380–383.

7. Chanfreau-Coffinier, Teutsch, and Fielding, "Assessing the Population Impact," https://nam.edu/wp-content/uploads/2015/06/PopulationImpactPublishedInterv entionStudies.pdf.

8. J. S. House, *Beyond Obamacare: Life, Death, and Social Policy* (New York: Russell Sage Foundation, 2015).

9. P. A. Briss, S. Zaza, M. Pappaioanou, et al., "Developing an Evidence-Based *Guide to Community Preventive Services*—Methods," *American Journal of Preventive Medicine* 18, suppl. 1 (2000): 35–43.

10. C. E. Steuerle, *Dead Men Ruling: How to Restore Fiscal Freedom and Rescue Our Future* (New York: Century Foundation Press, 2014).

11. L. M. Schwartz, S. Woloshin, F. J. Fowler Jr., and H. G. Welch, "Enthusiasm for Cancer Screening in the United States," *JAMA* 291 (2004): 71–78; L. M. Schwartz, S. Woloshin, and H. G. Welch, "Using a Drug Facts Box to Communicate Drug Benefits and Harms: Two Randomized Trials," *Annals of Internal Medicine* 150 (2009): 516–527.

12. H. Macdonald, "Navigating Uncertainty," *BJM* 357 (2017): j2524.

13. M. Baum, "'Catch It Early, Save a Life and Save a Breast': This Misleading Mantra of Mammography," *Journal of the Royal Society of Medicine* 108, no. 9 (2015): 338–339; R. F. Redberg and M. H. Katz, "Statins for Primary Prevention: The Debate Is Intense, but the Data Are Weak," *JAMA Internal Medicine* 177 (2017): 21–23.

14. V. Arora, C. Moriates, and N. Shah, *Understanding Value-Based Healthcare* (New York: McGraw Hill Professional, 2015).

15. R. Collins, C. Reith, J. Emberson, et al., "Interpretation of the Evidence for the Efficacy and Safety of Statin Therapy," *Lancet* 388 (2016): 2532–2561.

16. R. Knopp, M. d'Emden, J. Smilde, and S. Pocock, "Efficacy and Safety of Atorvastatin in the Prevention of Cardiovascular Endpoints in Subjects with Type 2 Diabetes: The Atorvastatin Study for Prevention of Coronary Heart Disease Endpoints in Non-Insulin-Dependent Diabetes Mellitus (ASPEN)," *Diabetes Care* 29, no. 7 (2006): 1478–1485.

17. J. R. Downs, M. Clearfield, S. Weis, et al., "Primary Prevention of Acute Coronary Events with Lovastatin in Men and Women with Average Cholesterol Levels: Results of AFCAPS/TexCAPS," *JAMA* 279, no. 20 (1998): 1615–1622.

18. M. F. Clarke, S. R. Quake, P. D. Dalerba, et al., "Methods and Systems for Analysis of Single Cells," US Patent 9,850,483, filed July 19, 2011, issued December 26, 2017.

19. J. E. Fielding, "Social Determinants of Health: Building Wide Coalitions around Well-Honed Messages," *American Journal of Public Health* 107 (2017): 870.

20. M. V. Maciosek, A. B. LaFrance, S. P. Dehmer, et al., "Updated Priorities among Effective Clinical Preventive Services," *Annals of Family Medicine* 15, no. 1 (2017): 14–22.

21. Redberg and Katz, "Statins for Primary Prevention"; J. P. Ioannidis, "Why Most Clinical Research Is Not Useful," *PLOS Medicine* 13 (2016): e1002049.

22. R. M. Kaplan and V. L. Irvin, "Likelihood of Null Effects of Large NHLBI Clinical Trials Has Increased over Time," *PLOS One* 10 (2015): e0132382.

23. W. Wan, "NIH Adopts New Rules on Human Research, Worrying Behavioral Scientists," *Washington Post,* January 24, 2018.

24. P. Lurie, H. S. Chahal, D. W. Sigelman, et al., "Comparison of Content of FDA Letters Not Approving Applications for New Drugs and Associated Public Announcements from Sponsors: Cross Sectional Study," *BMJ* 350 (2015): h2758.

25. J. Lenzer, *The Danger within Us: America's Untested, Unregulated Medical Device Industry and One Man's Battle to Survive It* (New York: Little Brown, 2017).

26. J. M. Sharfstein and M. Stebbins, "Enhancing Transparency at the US Food and Drug Administration: Moving Beyond the 21st Century Cures Act," *JAMA* 317, no. 16 (2017): 1621–1622.

27. N. Halfon, K. Larson, M. Lu, et al., "Lifecourse Health Development: Past, Present and Future," *Maternal and Child Health Journal* 18 (2014): 344–365.

28. C. A. Kiesler, "US Mental Health Policy: Doomed to Fail," *American Psychologist* 47 (1992): 1077–1082.

29. K. Larson, S. A. Russ, R. S. Kahn, et al., "Health Disparities: A Life Course Health Development Perspective and Future Research Directions," in *Handbook of Life Course Health Development,* ed. N. Halfon, C. Forrest, R. Lerner, and E. Faustman (Cham: Springer, 2018), 499–520..

30. N. Halfon, P. Long, D. I. Chang, et al., "Applying a 3.0 Transformation Framework to Guide Large-Scale Health System Reform," *Health Affairs* 33 (2014): 2003–2011.

31. N. Halfon, P. H. Wise, and C. B. Forrest, "The Changing Nature of Children's Health Development: New Challenges Require Major Policy Solutions," *Health Affairs* 33 (2014): 2116–2124.

32. A. Schickedanz, B. P. Dreyer, and N. Halfon, "Childhood Poverty: Understanding and Preventing the Adverse Impacts of a Most-Prevalent Risk to Pediatric Health and Well-Being," *Pediatric Clinics of North America* 62 (2015): 1111–1135.

33. G. P. Mays and S. A. Smith, "Evidence Links Increases in Public Health Spending to Declines in Preventable Deaths," *Health Affairs* 30, no. 8 (2011): 1585–1593.

34. J. D. Berry, A. Dyer, X. Cai, et al., "Lifetime Risks of Cardiovascular Disease," *NEJM* 366, no. 4 (2012): 321–329.

35. T.-H. T. Vu, M. R. Carnethon, K. Liu, et al., "Obesity Status in Younger Age, 39-Year Weight Change and Physical Performance in Older Age: The Chicago Healthy Aging Study (CHAS)," poster abstract, *Circulation* 135, suppl. 1 (2017): AP010.

36. J. Zissimopoulos, E. Crimmins, and P. St. Clair, "The Value of Delaying Alzheimer's Disease Onset," *Forum for Health Economics and Policy* 18, no. 1 (2014): 25–39.

37. "The 2016 Annual Homeless Assessment Report (AHAR) to Congress: Part 1, Point-in-Time Estimates of Homelessness," US Department of Housing and

Urban Development, Office of Community Planning and Development, Washington, DC, November 2016, https://www.hudexchange.info/resources /documents/2016-AHAR-Part-1.pdf.

38. M. H. Katz, "Homelessness—Challenges and Progress," *JAMA* 318, no. 23 (2017): 2293–2294.

39. T. P. Baggett, S. W. Hwang, J. J. O'Connell, et al., "Mortality among Homeless Adults in Boston: Shifts in Causes of Death over a 15-Year Period," *JAMA Internal Medicine* 173, no.3 (2013): 189–195.

40. P. Reilly, "Why Hawaii Bill Would Treat Homelessness as a Medical Condition," *Christian Science Monitor,* January 27, 2017.

41. Helping Hands Hawaiʻi, 2015 Annual Report, http://helpinghandshawaii.org/wp -content/uploads/HHH-Annual-Report-2015FINAL.compressed.pdf.

42. M. Sandel and M. Desmond, "Investing in Housing for Health Improves Both Mission and Margin," *JAMA* 318, no. 23 (2017): 2291–2292.

43. A. L. Brewster, S. Kunkel, J. Straker, and L. A. Curry, "Cross-Sectoral Partnerships by Area Agencies on Aging: Associations with Health Care Use and Spending," *Health Affairs* 37 (2018): 15–21.

44. Brewster, Kunkel, Straker, and Curry, "Cross-Sectoral Partnerships"; K. Armstrong, "Chemobrain: Physiological Predisposing Factors," *Medsurg Nursing* 25, no. 4 (2016): 215–218.

45. S. L. Szanton, Y. N. Alfonso, B. Leff, et al., "Medicaid Cost Savings of a Preventive Home Visit Program for Disabled Older Adults," *Journal of the American Geriatrics Society* 66, no. 3 (2018): 614–620.

46. T. R. Frieden, K. Ethier, and A. Schuchat, "Improving the Health of the United States with a 'Winnable Battles' Initiative," *JAMA* 317, no. 9 (2017): 903–904.

47. L. W. Green, J. M. Ottoson, C. García, and R. A. Hiatt, "Diffusion Theory and Knowledge Dissemination, Utilization, and Integration in Public Health," *Annual Review of Public Health* 30 (2009): 151–174.

48. R. C. Brownson, G. A. Colditz, and E. K. Proctor, *Dissemination and Implementation Research in Health: Translating Science to Practice* (New York: Oxford University Press, 2012).

49. "The All of Us Research Program," website, National Institutes of Health, https://allofus.nih.gov/.

50. S. H. Woolf and L. Y. Aron, "The US Health Disadvantage Relative to Other High-Income Countries: Findings from a National Research Council / Institute of Medicine Report," *JAMA* 309, no. 8 (2013): 771–772.

51. Institute of Medicine, Committee on the Learning Health Care System in America, *Best Care at Lower Cost: The Path to Continuously Learning Health Care in America,* ed. M. Smith, R. Saunders, L. Stuckhardt, and J. M. McGinnis (Washington, DC: National Academies Press, 2013).

52. D. M. Berwick and A. D. Hackbarth, "Eliminating Waste in US Health Care," *JAMA* 307 (2012): 1513–1516.

53. R. J. Reid and E. H. Wagner, "The Veterans Health Administration Patient Aligned Care Teams: Lessons in Primary Care Transformation," *Journal of General Internal Medicine* 29, suppl. 2 (2014): S552–S554.

54. R. M. Kaplan, *Disease, Diagnoses, and Dollars* (New York: Springer, 2009).
55. A. McPhee, A. Ali, H. Rush, and G. Oades, "Small Renal Mass Biopsies: An Effective Tool in Avoiding Unnecessary Surgery," *European Journal of Cancer* 72, suppl. 1 (2017): S189–S190; B. E. Jones and M. H. Samore, "Antibiotic Overuse: Clinicians Are the Solution," *Annals of Internal Medicine* 166 (2017): 844–845.
56. V. Saini, S. Garcia-Armesto, D. Klemperer, et al., "Drivers of Poor Medical Care," *Lancet* 390 (2017): 178–190.
57. S. T. Rinne, A. J. Walkey, M.-S. Shieh, et al., "Regional Variation in Do Not Resuscitate Orders and End of Life Health Care Use and Spending in the United States," abstract, *American Journal of Respiratory and Critical Care Medicine* 195 (2017): A7099.
58. L. P. Casalino, D. Gans, R. Weber, et al., "US Physician Practices Spend More than $15.4 Billion Annually to Report Quality Measures," *Health Affairs* 35 (2016): 401–406.
59. D. M. Berwick, "Era 3 for Medicine and Health Care," *JAMA* 315 (2016): 1329–1330.
60. T. Rice, P. Rosenau, L. Y. Unruh, and A. J. Barnes, "United States of America: Health System Review," *Health Systems in Transition* 15, no. 3 (2013), http://www.euro.who.int/__data/assets/pdf_file/0019/215155/HiT-United-States -of-America.pdf.
61. S. Brill, *America's Bitter Pill: Money, Politics, Backroom Deals, and the Fight to Fix Our Broken Healthcare System* (New York: Random House, 2015).
62. T. Rice, *The Economics of Health Reconsidered* (Chicago: Health Administration Press, 1998).
63. M. L. Spittel, W. T. Riley, and R. M. Kaplan, "Educational Attainment and Life Expectancy: A Perspective from the NIH Office of Behavioral and Social Sciences Research," *Social Science and Medicine* 127 (2015): 203–205.

Appendix

1. A. C. Heath, K. M. Kirk, J. M. Meyer, and N. G. Martin, "Genetic and Social Determinants of Initiation and Age at Onset of Smoking in Australian Twins," *Behavioral Genetics* 29 (1999): 395–407; H. H. Maes, M. C. Neale, K. S. Kendler, et al. "Genetic and Cultural Transmission of Smoking Initiation: An Extended Twin Kinship Model," *Behavioral Genetics* 36 (2006): 795–808; A. Agrawal, P. A. Madden, A. C. Heath, et al., "Correlates of Regular Cigarette Smoking in a Population-Based Sample of Australian Twins," *Addiction* 100 (2005): 1709–1719; P. A. Madden, A. C. Heath, N. L. Pedersen, et al., "The Genetics of Smoking Persistence in Men and Women: A Multicultural Study," *Behavioral Genetics* 29 (1999): 423–431.
2. L. Perusse, A. Tremblay, C. Leblanc, et al., "Familial Resemblance in Energy Intake: Contribution of Genetic and Environmental Factors," *American Journal of Clinical Nutrition* 47 (1988): 629–635; D. R. Reed, A. A. Bachmanov, G. K. Beauchamp et al., "Heritable Variation in Food Preferences and Their Contribution to Obesity," *Behavioral Genetics* 27 (1997): 373–387.

3. K. Samaras, P. J. Kelly, M. N. Chiano, et al., "Genetic and Environmental Influ-
    ences on Total-Body and Central Abdominal Fat: The Effect of Physical
    Activity in Female Twins," *Annals of Internal Medicine* 130 (1999): 873–882.
4. F. Ducci, M. A. Enoch, C. Hodgkinson, et al., "Interaction between a
    Functional MAOA Locus and Childhood Sexual Abuse Predicts Alcoholism
    and Antisocial Personality Disorder in Adult Women," *Molecular Psychiatry*
    13 (2008): 334–347.
5. R. B. Williams, "Lower Central Nervous System Serotonergic Function and
    Risk of Cardiovascular Disease: Where Are We, What's Next?" *Stroke* 38
    (2007): 2213–2214.
6. D. Ornish, M. J. Magbanua, G. Weidner, et al., "Changes in Prostate Gene
    Expression in Men Undergoing an Intensive Nutrition and Lifestyle Interven-
    tion," *PNAS* 105 (2008): 8369–8374.
7. J. P. Capitanio, K. Abel, S. P. Mendoza, et al., "Personality and Serotonin
    Transporter Genotype Interact with Social Context to Affect Immunity and
    Viral Set-Point in Simian Immunodeficiency Virus Disease," *Brain, Behavior,
    and Immunity* 22 (2008): 676–689.
8. Centers for Disease Control and Prevention, *The Health Consequences of
    Smoking: A Report of the Surgeon General* (Atlanta: US Department of Health
    and Human Services, CDC, 2004).
9. M. Sharma, "Behavioural Interventions for Preventing and Treating Obesity in
    Adults," *Obesity Reviews* 8 (2007): 441–449; US Department of Health and
    Human Services, *The Surgeon General's Call to Action to Prevent and
    Decrease Overweight and Obesity* (Washington, DC: Public Health Service,
    Office of the Surgeon General, 2001); A. Must, J. Spadano, E. H. Coakley, et al.,
    "The Disease Burden Associated with Overweight and Obesity," *JAMA* 282
    (1999): 1523–1529; National Heart, Lung, and Blood Institute and National
    Institute of Diabetes and Digestive and Kidney Disease, *Clinical Guidelines on
    the Identification, Evaluation, and Treatment of Overweight and Obesity in
    Adults,* report no. 98–4083 (Washington, DC: National Institutes of Health,
    1998); E. E. Calle and M. J. Thun, "Obesity and Cancer," *Oncogene* 23 (2004):
    6365–6378; J. H. Goldberg and A. C. King, "Physical Activity and Weight
    Management across the Lifespan," *Annual Review of Public Health* 28 (2007):
    145–170; M. B. Schulze and F. B. Hu, "Primary Prevention of Diabetes: What
    Can Be Done and How Much Can Be Prevented?" *Annual Review of Public
    Health* 26 (2005): 445–467.
10. S. N. Blair, H. W. Kohl III, R. S. Paffenbarger Jr.,et al., "Physical Fitness and
    All-Cause Mortality: A Prospective Study of Healthy Men and Women," *JAMA*
    262 (1989): 2395–2401.
11. W. L. Haskell, I. M. Lee, R. R. Pate, et al., "Physical Activity and Public Health:
    Updated Recommendation for Adults from the American College of Sports
    Medicine and the American Heart Association," *Medicine and Science in Sports
    and Exercise* 39 (2007):1423–1434; J. A. Berlin and G. A. Colditz, "A Meta-
    Analysis of Physical Activity in the Prevention of Coronary Heart Disease,"
    American Journal of Epidemiology 132 (1990): 612–628; K. E. Powell, P. D.
    Thompson, C. J. Caspersen, and J. S. Kendrick, "Physical Activity and the

Incidence of Coronary Heart Disease," *Annual Review of Public Health* 8 (1987)8: 253–287.

12. Healthy People 2010. Leading Health Indicators 2000, https://healthypeople.gov /2010/LHI/.

13. R. H. Eckel and R. M. Krauss, for the AHA Nutrition Committee, "American Heart Association Call to Action: Obesity as a Major Risk Factor for Coronary Heart Disease," *Circulation* 97 (1998): 2099–2100.

14. Office of Behavioral and Social Sciences Research, *The Contributions of Behavioral and Social Sciences Research to Improving the Health of the Nation: A Prospectus for the Future* (Washington, DC: U.S. Department of Health and Human Services, National Institutes of Health, August 2007); L. H. Kuller, "Dietary Fat and Chronic Diseases: Epidemiologic Overview," *Journal of the American Dietetic Association* 97 (1997): S9-S15; P. Greenwald, C. K. Clifford, and J. A. Milner, "Diet and Cancer Prevention," *European Journal of Cancer* 37 (2001): 948–965; B. Rockhill, W. C. Willett, D. J. Hunter, et al., "A Prospective Study of Recreational Physical Activity and Breast Cancer Risk," *Archives of Internal Medicine* 159 (1999): 2290–2296; C. E. Matthews, X. O. Shu, F. Jin, et al., "Lifetime Physical Activity and Breast Cancer Risk in the Shanghai Breast Cancer Study," *British Journal of Cancer* 84 (2001): 994–1001; I. Thune, T. Brenn, E. Lund, and M. Gaard, "Physical Activity and the Risk of Breast Cancer," *NEJM* 1997 (336): 1269–1275.

15. E. M. Reiche, S. O. Nunes, and H. K. Morimoto, "Stress, Depression, the Immune System, and Cancer," *Lancet Oncology* 5 (2004): 617–625; J. Leserman, "Role of Depression, Stress, and Trauma in HIV Disease Progression," *Psychosomatic Medicine* 70 (2008): 539–545.

16. N. R. Anthonisen, M. A. Skeans, R. A. Wise, et al., "The Effects of a Smoking Cessation Intervention on 14.5-Year Mortality: A Randomized Clinical Trial," *Annals of Internal Medicine* 142 (2005): 233–239.

17. K. J. Campbell and K. D. Hesketh, "Strategies Which Aim to Positively Impact on Weight, Physical Activity, Diet and Sedentary Behaviours in Children from Zero to Five Years: A Systematic Review of the Literature," *Obesity Reviews* 8 (2007): 327–338; C. D. Summerbell, E. Waters, L. D. Edmunds, et al., "Interventions for Preventing Obesity in Children," *Cochrane Database of Systematic Reviews* (2005): CD001871; L. H. Epstein, A. Valoski, R. R. Wing, and J. McCurley, "Ten-Year Outcomes of Behavioral Family-Based Treatment for Childhood Obesity," *Health Psychology* 13 (1994): 373–383; M. L. Fitzgibbon, M. R. Stolley, L. Schiffer, et al., "Two-Year Follow-Up Results for Hip-Hop to Health Jr.: A Randomized Controlled Trial for Overweight Prevention in Preschool Minority Children," *Journal of Pediatrics* 146 (2005): 618–625; J. B. Connelly, M. J. Duaso, and G. Butler, "A Systematic Review of Controlled Trials of Interventions to Prevent Childhood Obesity and Overweight: A Realistic Synthesis of the Evidence," *Public Health* 121 (2007): 510–517; L. DeMattia, L. Lemont, and L. Meurer, "Do Interventions to Limit Sedentary Behaviours Change Behaviour and Reduce Childhood Obesity? A Critical Review of the Literature," *Obesity Reviews* 8 (2007): 69–81.

18. M. Savoye, M. Shaw, J. Dziura, et al., "Effects of a Weight Management Program on Body Composition and Metabolic Parameters in Overweight Children," *JAMA* 297 (2007): 2697–2704.

19. A. Swartz, S. Strath, D. Bassett, et al. "Increasing Daily Walking Improves Glucose Tolerance in Overweight Women," *Preventive Medicine* 37 (2003): 356–362.

20. M. J. O'Connor and S. E. Whaley, "Brief Intervention for Alcohol Use by Pregnant Women," *American Journal of Public Health* 97 (2007): 252–258.

21. Diabetes Prevention Program Research Group, "Reduction of the Incidence of Type 2 Diabetes with Lifestyle Intervention or Metformin," *NEJM* 346 (2002): 393–403; J. Tuomilehto, J. Lindstrom, J. G. Ericksson, et al., "Prevention of Type 2 Diabetes Mellitus by Changes in Lifestyle among Subjects with Impaired Glucose Tolerance," *NEJM* 344 (2001): 1343–1350; J. Lindstrom, P. Ilanne-Parikka, M. Peltonen, et al., "Sustained Reduction in the Incidence of Type 2 Diabetes by Lifestyle Intervention: Follow-Up of the Finnish Diabetes Prevention Study," *Lancet* 368 (2006): 1673–1679.

22. J. A. Meyerhardt, D. Heseltine, D. Niedzwiecki, et al., "Impact of Physical Activity on Cancer Recurrence and Survival in Patients with Stage III Colon Cancer: Findings from CALGB 89803," *Journal of Clinical Oncology* 24 (2006): 3535–3541; A. K. Samad, R. S. Taylor, T. Marshall, and M. A. Chapman, "A Meta-Analysis of the Association of Physical Activity with Reduced Risk of Colorectal Cancer," *Colorectal Disease* 7 (2005): 204–213; R. Ballard-Barbash, A. Schatzkin, D. Albanes, et al., "Physical Activity and Risk of Large Bowel Cancer in the Framingham Study," *Cancer Research* 50 (1990): 3610–3613; M. E. Martinez, E. Giovannucci, D. Spiegelman, et al., "Leisure-Time Physical Activity, Body Size, and Colon Cancer in Women," *Journal of the National Cancer Institute* 89 (1997): 948–955; I. M. Lee, R. S. Paffenbarger Jr., and C. Hsieh, "Physical Activity and Risk of Developing Colorectal Cancer among College Alumni," *Journal of the National Cancer Institute* 83 (1991): 1324–1329; D. Albanes, A. Blair, and P. R. Taylor, "Physical Activity and Risk of Cancer in the NHANES I Population," *American Journal of Public Health* 79 (1989): 744–750; M. J. Thun, E. E. Calle, M. M. Namboodiri, et al., "Risk Factors for Fatal Colon Cancer in a Large Prospective Study," *Journal of the National Cancer Institute* 84 (1992): 1491–1500.

23. US Preventive Services Task Force, "Behavioral Counseling to Prevent Sexually Transmitted Infections: U.S. Preventive Services Task Force Recommendation Statement," *Annals of Internal Medicine* 149, no. 7 (2008): 491–496.

24. M. C. Fiore, W. C. Bailey, S. J. Cohen, et al., *Treating Tobacco Use and Dependence: Clinical Practice Guideline* (Rockville, MD: US Dept. of Health and Human Services, Public Health Service, 2000).

25. R. Perez-Escamilla, A. Hromi-Fiedler, S. Vega-Lopez, et al., "Impact of Peer Nutrition Education on Dietary Behaviors and Health Outcomes among Latinos: A Systematic Literature Review," *Journal of Nutrition Education and Behavior* 40 (2008): 208–225.

26. N. G. Boule, E. Haddad, G. P. Kenny, et al., "Effects of Exercise on Glycemic Control and Body Mass in Type 2 Diabetes Mellitus: A Meta-Analysis of Controlled Clinical Trials," *JAMA* 286 (2001): 1218–1227.

27. US Preventive Services Task Force, "Screening and Behavioral Counseling Inverventions in Primary Care to Reduce Alcohol Misuse: Recommendation Statement," *American Family Physician* 70, no. 2 (2004): 353–358; E. P. Whitlock, M. R. Polen, C. A. Green, et al., "Behavioral Counseling Interventions in Primary Care to Reduce Risky / Harmful Alcohol Use by Adults: A Summary of the Evidence for the U.S. Preventive Services Task Force," *Annals of Internal Medicine* 140 (2004): 557–568.

28. S. L. Norris, M. M. Engelgau, and K. M. Narayan, "Effectiveness of Self-Management Training in Type 2 Diabetes: A Systematic Review of Randomized Controlled Trials," *Diabetes Care* 24 (2001): 561–587.

29. S. L. Norris, J. Lau, S. J. Smith, et al., "Self-Management Education for Adults with Type 2 Diabetes: A Meta-Analysis of the Effect on Glycemic Control," *Diabetes Care* 25 (2002): 1159–1171; R. M. Anderson, M. M. Funnell, P. A. Barr, et al., "Learning to Empower Patients: Results of Professional Education Program for Diabetes Educators," *Diabetes Care* 14 (1991): 584–590; R. M. Anderson, M. M. Funnell, P. M. Butler, et al., "Patient Empowerment: Results of a Randomized Controlled Trial," *Diabetes Care* 18 (1995): 943–949; S. Greenfield, S. H. Kaplan, J. E. Ware, et al., "Patients' Participation in Medical Care: Effects on Blood Sugar Control and Quality of Life in Diabetes," *Journal of General Internal Medicine* 3 (1988): 448–457; R. R. Rubin, M. Peyrot, and C. D. Saudek, "Effect of Diabetes Education on Self-Care, Metabolic Control, and Emotional Well-Being," *Diabetes Care* 12 (1989): 673–679; R. R. Rubin, M. Peyrot, and C. D. Saudek, "The Effect of a Comprehensive Diabetes Education Program Incorporating Coping Skills Training on Emotional Wellbeing and Diabetes Self-Efficacy," *Diabetes Educator* 19 (1993): 210–214; I. Muhlhauser and M. Berger, "Diabetes Education and Insulin Therapy: When Will They Ever Learn?" *Journal of Internal Medicine* 233 (1993): 321–326; T. R. Pieber, G. A. Brunner, W. J. Schnedl, et al., "Evaluation of a Structured Outpatient Group Education Program for Intensive Insulin Therapy," *Diabetes Care* 18 (1995): 625–630; S. Clement, "Diabetes Self-Management Education," *Diabetes Care* 18 (1995): 1204–1214; R. E. Aubert, W. H. Herman, J. Waters, et al., "Nurse Case Management to Improve Glycemic Control in Diabetic Patients in a Health Maintenance Organization: A Randomized, Controlled Trial," *Annals of Internal Medicine* 129 (1998): 605–612.

30. R. Glasgow, D. J. Toobert, and S. Hampson, "Participation in Outpatient Diabetes Education Programs: How Many Patients Take Part and How Representative Are They?" *Diabetes Educator* 5 (1991): 376–380; R. E. Glasgow, D. J. Toobert, S. E. Hampson, et al., "Improving Self-Care among Older Patients with Type II Diabetes: The 'Sixty Something . . .' Study," *Patient Education and Counseling* 19 (1992): 61–74; R. M. Anderson, W. H. Herman, J. M. Davis, et al., "Barriers to Improving Diabetes Care for Black Persons," *Diabetes Care* 14 (1991): 605–609.

31. The Diabetes Control and Complications Trial Research Group, "The Effect of Intensive Treatment of Diabetes on the Development and Progression of Long-Term Complications in Insulin-Dependent Diabetes Mellitus," *NEJM* 329 (1993): 977–986; The Diabetes Control and Complications Trial

Research Group, "Implementation of Treatment Protocols in the Diabetes Control and Complications Trial," *Diabetes Care* 18 (1995): 361–376.

32. The Diabetes Control and Complications Trial/Epidemiology of Diabetes Interventions and Complications (DCCT/EDIC) Study Research Group, "Intensive Diabetes Treatment and Cardiovascular Disease in Patients with Type 1 Diabetes," *NEJM* 353 (2005): 2643–2653.

33. D. Ornish, L. W. Scherwitz, J. H. Billings, et al., "Intensive Lifestyle Changes for Reversal of Coronary Heart Disease," *JAMA* 280 (1998): 2001–2007.

34. G. C. Fonarow, A. Gawlinski, S. Moughrabi, and J. Tillisch, "Improved Treatment of Coronary Heart Disease by Implementation of a Cardiac Hospitalization Atherosclerosis Management Program (CHAMP)," *American Journal of Cardiology* 87 (2001): 819–822.

35. M. G. MacVicar, M. L. Winningham, and J. L. Nickel, "Effects of Aerobic Interval Training on Cancer Patients' Functional Capacity," *Nursing Research* 38 (1989): 348–351; F. Dimeo, S. Fetscher, W. Lange, et al., "Effects of Aerobic Exercise on the Physical Performance and Incidence of Treatment-Related Complications after High-Dose Chemotherapy," *Blood* 90 (1997): 3390–3394; V. Mock, K. H. Dow, C. J. Meares, et al. "Effects of Exercise on Fatigue, Physical Functioning, and Emotional Distress during Radiation Therapy for Breast Cancer," *Oncology Nursing Forum* 24 (1997): 991–1000.

36. Office of Behavioral and Social Sciences Research, *The Contributions of Behavioral and Social Sciences Research to Improving the Health of the Nation: A Prospectus for the Future* (Washington, DC: US Department of Health and Human Services, National Institutes of Health, August 2007).

37. D. Wilson, J. Parsons, and M. Wakefield, "The Health-Related Quality-of-Life of Never Smokers, Ex-Smokers, and Light, Moderate, and Heavy Smokers," *Preventive Medicine* 29 (1999): 139–144; T. Ostbye and D. H. Taylor, "The Effect of Smoking on Years of Healthy Life (YHL) Lost among Middle-Aged and Older Americans," *Health Services Research* 39 (2004): 531–552; K. Crothers, T. A. Griffith, K. A. McGinnis, et al., "The Impact of Cigarette Smoking on Mortality, Quality of Life, and Comorbid Illness among HIV-Positive Veterans," *Journal of General Internal Medicine* 20 (2005): 1142–1145; Y. I. Garces, P. Yang, J. Parkinson, et al., "The Relationship between Cigarette Smoking and Quality of Life after Lung Cancer Diagnosis," *Chest* 126 (2004): 1733–1741.

38. A. Drewnowski and W. J. Evans, "Nutrition, Physical Activity, and Quality of Life in Older Adults: Summary," *Journals of Gerontology,* series a, 56 suppl. 2 (2001): 89–94; M. F. Scheier, V. S. Helgeson, R. Schulz, et al., "Interventions to Enhance Physical and Psychological Functioning among Younger Women Who Are Ending Nonhormonal Adjuvant Treatment for Early-Stage Breast Cancer," *Journal of Clinical Oncology* 23 (2005): 4298–4311; K. R. Fontaine and I. Barofsky, "Obesity and Health-Related Quality of Life," *Obesity Reviews* 2 (2001): 173–182.

39. Drewnowski and Evans, "Nutrition, Physical Activity, and Quality of Life"; W. J. Rejeski, L. R. Brawley, and S. A. Shumaker, "Physical Activity and Health-Related Quality of Life," *Exercise and Sport Sciences Reviews* 24 (1996): 71–108.

40. K. S. Courneya, "Exercise in Cancer Survivors: An Overview of Research," *Medicine and Science in Sports and Exercise* 35 (2003): 1846–1852.

41. J. T. Arnedt, D. Conroy, J. Rutt, et al., "An Open Trial of Cognitive-Behavioral Treatment for Insomnia Comorbid with Alcohol Dependence," *Sleep Medicine* 8 (2007): 176–180.

42. J. Blumenthal, A. Sherwood, M. Babyak, et al., "Effects of Exercise and Stress Management Training on Markers of Cardiovascular Risk in Patients with Ischemic Heart Disease," *JAMA* 293 (2005): 1626–1634.

43. J. Castaldo and J. Reed, "The Lowering of Vascular Atherosclerotic Risk (LOVAR) Program: An Approach to Modifying Cerebral, Cardiac, and Peripheral Vascular Disease," *Journal of Stroke and Cerebrovascular Diseases* 17 (2008): 9–15.

44. M. J. Vale, M. V. Jelinek, J. D. Best, et al., "Coaching Patients on Achieving Cardiovascular Health (COACH): A Multicenter Randomized Trial in Patients with Coronary Heart Disease," *Archives of Internal Medicine* 163 (2003): 2775–2783.

45. P. Ades, F. Pashkow, G. Fletcher, et al., "A Controlled Trial of Cardiac Rehabilitation in the Home Setting Using Electrocardiographic and Voice Transtelephonic Monitoring," *American Heart Journal* 139 (2000): 543–548; J. Cochran and V. S. Conn, "Meta-Analysis of Quality of Life Outcomes Following Diabetes Self-Management Training," *Diabetes Educator* 34 (2008): 815–823; L. Lalonde, K. Gray-Donald, I. Lowensteyn, et al., "Comparing the Benefits of Diet and Exercise in the Treatment of Dyslipidemia," *Preventive Medicine* 35 (2002): 16–24; C. M. Yu, L. S. Li, H. H. Ho, and C. P. Lau, "Long-Term Changes in Exercise Capacity, Quality of Life, Body Anthropometry, and Lipid Profiles after a Cardiac Rehabilitation Program in Obese Patients with Coronary Heart Disease," *American Journal of Cardiology* 91 (2003): 321–325.

46. M. H. Antoni, J. M. Lehman, K. M. Kilbourn, et al., "Cognitive-Behavioral Stress Management Intervention Decreases the Prevalence of Depression and Enhances Benefit Finding among Women under Treatment for Early-Stage Breast Cancer," *Health Psychology* 20 (2001): 20–32; S. J. Lepore, V. S. Helgeson, D. T. Eton, and R. Schulz, "Improving Quality of Life in Men with Prostate Cancer: A Randomized Controlled Trial of Group Education Interventions," *Health Psychology* 22 (2003): 443–452; M. A. Lieberman, M. Golant, J. Giese-Davis, et al., "Electronic Support Groups for Breast Carcinoma: A Clinical Trial of Effectiveness," *Cancer* 97 (2003): 920–925; F. J. Penedo, J. R. Dahn, I. Molton, et al., "Cognitive-Behavioral Stress Management Improves Stress-Management Skills and Quality of Life in Men Recovering from Treatment of Prostate Carcinoma," *Cancer* 100 (2004): 192–200.

47. M. H. Antoni, A. Caricco, R. Duran, et al., "Randomized Clinical Trial of Cognitive Behavioral Stress Management on HIV Viral Load in Gay Men Treated with HAART," *Psychosomatic Medicine* 68 (2006): 143–151; L. A. Scott-Sheldon, S. C. Kalichman, M. P. Carey, and R. L. Fielder, "Stress Management Interventions for HIV+ Adults: A Meta-Analysis of Randomized Controlled Trials, 1989 to 2006," *Health Psychology* 27 (2008): 129–139.

48. C. M. Fichtenberg and S. A. Glantz, "Association of the California Tobacco Control Program with Declines in Cigarette Consumption and Mortality from Heart Disease," *NEJM* 343 (2000): 1772–1777.

49. A. Jemal, M. J. Thun, and L. A. Ries, et al., "Annual Report to the Nation on the Status of Cancer, 1975–2005, Featuring Trends in Lung Cancer, Tobacco Use, and Tobacco Control," *Journal of the National Cancer Institute* 100 (2008): 1672–1694.

50. M. P. Stern, J. W. Farquhar, N. McCoby, and S. H. Russell, "Results of a Two-Year Health Education Campaign on Dietary Behavior: The Stanford Three Community Study," *Circulation* 54 (1976): 826–833.

51. A. McAlister, P. Puska, J. T. Salonen, et al., "Theory and Action for Health Promotion Illustrations from the North Karelia Project," *American Journal of Public Health* 72 (1982) :43–50; P. Puska, A. Nissinen, J. Tuomilehto, et al., "The Community-Based Strategy to Prevent Coronary Heart Disease: Conclusions from the Ten Years of the North Karelia Project," *Annual Review of Public Health* 6 (1985): 147–193.

52. C. E. Staunton, D. Hubsmith, and W. Kallins, "Promoting Safe Walking and Biking to School: The Marin County Success Story," *American Journal of Public Health* 93 (2003): 1431–1434; R. C. Brownson, R. A. Housemann, D. R. Brown, et al., "Promoting Physical Activity in Rural Communities: Walking Trail Access, Use, and Effects," *American Journal of Preventive Medicine* 18 (2000): 235–241.

53. Centers for Disease Control and Prevention, *Preventing Excessive Alcohol Use,* CDC fact sheet, https://www.cdc.gov/alcohol/fact-sheets/prevention.htm.

acknowledgments

The original manuscript for this book was nearly twice its current length, so shortening it to the book you hold in your hands was a challenge. Equally difficult is expressing my deepest thanks to all who have contributed to the book without risking a return to its previous length. I was aided by two fellowships, beginning with one from the Center for Advanced Study in the Behavioral Sciences at Stanford University, where I had the opportunity to think, reflect, and write. There, in one of the most beautiful settings imaginable, I was surrounded by cherished colleagues and friends. I am particularly indebted to center director Margaret Levy and her staff, and Michael Gaetani's repeated inquiries, "When is that book going to be done?" did serve a purpose. Louis Hyman read an early version and suggested that Harvard University Press would be the right publisher. Many colleagues at the center, including Marty Gilens, Victor Quintanilla, and Dan Rodgers, sacrificed lunch hours to guide my thinking. Adam Minor read the entire first draft and offered many insightful comments, and Lynda Powell served as a regular sounding board and mentor.

The book was finished in 2018 while I was a resident scholar at the Rockefeller Foundation Bellagio Center on Lake Como in Italy. This term was a capstone of support for a long career and abiding interest in public health, and I hope I have honored the foundation's mission of merging the thoughts, ideas, and talents of fellows past and present. I am particularly indebted to director Pilar Palacia and her superb staff for creating the best work environment imaginable. Many colleagues from the center made substantive contributions, including Bob Barsky, Arthur Blume, Jody Hyman, Marcia Linn, Jonatas Manzolli, Dikgang Moseneke, Mshai Mwangola, Katie Redford, Jan Schaffer, and Karen Schmaling.

My view of health and health care was evolving as I entered government service as the director of the Office of Behavioral and Social Sciences Research at the National Institutes of Health and later as chief science officer at the Agency for Healthcare Research and Quality. My years at NIH gave me exposure to both the promise and the limitations of biomedical research, and also the benefit of working closely with Stephane Philogene, Deb Olster, and Mike Spittel on some of the nation's most pressing health issues. David Chambers, Bob Croyle, and Russ Glasgow from the National Cancer Institute had a very important influence on the early development of this book. Veronica Irvin collaborated on the work that led me to rethink the expected outcomes of large clinical trials. AHRQ director Rick Kronick repeatedly used his razor-sharp intellect to identify arguments that needed clarification or rethinking. Other AHRQ colleagues, including Sharon Arnold, David Meyers, and Jason Sutherland, also contributed to the journey.

For nearly a quarter century, I have been a member of the teaching faculty for the American Heart Association Seminar on the Epidemiology and Prevention of Cardiovascular Disease and Stroke. The fellows, who represent the best and brightest of young physicians and public health scientists, taught me more than I taught them, and many of these lessons found their way into the manuscript. To my Tahoe faculty colleagues, including Cheryl Anderson, Alain Bertoni, Mike Criqui, Henry Feldman, David Goff, Kathy Grady, George Howard, Fleetwood Loustalot, and Darwin Labarthe, thanks for listening.

As the book progressed, I have been fortunate to work with Arnold Milstein, director of the Clinical Excellence Research Center at Stanford University, who has been an important mentor and role model. Arnie gave me the space to get the manuscript out the door. Stanford colleagues Steve Ash, Alan Glaseroff, Jill Glassman, Craig Lindquist, and Claude Pinnock have been attentive listeners and helpful sounding boards.

Over the last two years, I was given the opportunity to be a grand rounds or colloquium speaker at Boston University, Northwestern University, the University of Michigan, Purdue University, Stanford University, the University of California–Riverside, the University of Southern California, the National Academy of Medicine, and the University of Toronto's Hospital for Sick Children. With feedback from the audiences at these universities, the manuscript evolved. Similar appreciation is owed to my colleagues at UCLA and UCSD, where I have continuing collaborations. And I owe a particular debt to Dawn Wilson and Terry Cronan for their ongoing interest and support of this work.

In addition to the multiple anonymous peer reviewers, Bonnie Spring from Northwestern University and Howard Friedman from the University of California–Riverside read and critiqued sections of the manuscript.

I am particularly indebted to the dedicated and talented staff at Harvard University Press for making this book possible. Janice Audet, my editor, has been a tireless advocate. Although I have completed previous book projects, I have never had an editor with Janice's depth of knowledge and expertise. She read and edited all versions of the manuscript, provided guidance, and attended to every detail. Janice is that rare combination of smart, supportive, highly competent, and efficient; I feel fortunate to have had the chance to work with her. Simon Waxman, an exceptionally talented editor, helped completely reshape a much longer and less focused manuscript. He was patient and extremely skillful in finding a pathway to conciseness. Special thanks to senior production editor Melody Negron, from Westchester Publishing Services, and editorial assistant Esther Blanco Benmaman, intellectual property director Stephanie Vyce, and senior editor Louise Robbins from Harvard University Press. The production crew at Harvard University Press and Westchester Publishing Services dealt expertly with edits and the inclusion of new studies, and they did a fantastic job of keeping the book moving forward.

We are a public health family, and even family events often include discussions about the future of health care and biomedical research. It started with my father, Dr. Oscar Kaplan, and continues with my kids, Dr. Cameron Kaplan from the University of Southern California, Seth Kaplan from HonorHealth in Scottsdale, and Ashley Pye from Hollywood Presbyterian Medical Center.

Finally, my wife, Margaret Gaston, lived with the project from the beginning. As my most supportive critic, she helped me say what I wanted to say, while helping me avoid saying what I shouldn't. Margaret feels the weighty responsibility of keeping me on track while maintaining life balance. As always, it worked.

credits

Figure 1.1. Reproduced from R. M. Kaplan, D. H. David, and M. L. Spittel, "Innovations in Population Health Research: The Challenge," in *Population Health: Behavioral and Social Science Insights,* ed. R. M. Kaplan, M. L. Spittel, and D. H. David, AHRQ Publication No. 15–0002 (Rockville, MD: Agency for Healthcare Research and Quality and Office of Behavioral and Social Sciences Research, National Institutes of Health, 2015), p. 2.

Figure 1.2. *US Health in International Perspective: Shorter Lives, Poorer Health* (Washington, DC: National Academies Press, 2013), figs. 1.7 and 1.8. Reproduced by permission of the National Academies Press.

Figure 3.1. Adapted from W. B. Kannel, M. J. Garcia, P. M. McNamara, et al., "Serum Lipid Precursors of Coronary Heart Disease," *Human Pathology* 2.1 (1971), fig. 3.

Figure 3.2. Adapted from R. M. Kaplan, "Physicians' Health Study: Aspirin and Primary Prevention of Heart Disease," Letter to the Editor, *New England Journal of Medicine* 321 (1989): 1825–1828.

Figure 3.3. Adapted from Action to Control Cardiovascular Risk in Diabetes Study Group (H. C. Gerstein, M. E. Miller, et al.), "Effects of Intensive Glucose Lowering in Type 2 Diabetes," *New England Journal of Medicine* 358 (2008): 2545–2559, fig. 1 (p. 2550).

Figure 5.1. Reproduced with permission from Virginia Commonwealth University Center on Society and Health.

Figure 5.2. Adapted from R. Wilkinson and K. Pickett, *The Spirit Level: Why Greater Equality Makes Societies Stronger* (New York: Bloomsbury Press, 2009), fig. 2.2, by permission of the authors.

Figure 5.3. Data source: for blood pressure, diabetes, employment, smoking, and cholesterol, estimated from R. Clarke, J. Emberson,

A. Fletcher, et al., "Life Expectancy in Relation to Cardiovascular Risk Factors: 38 Year Follow-up of 19,000 Men in the Whitehall Study," *BMJ* 339 (2009): b3513; for living environment, courtesy of Steven Woolf, Virginia Commonwealth University.

Figure 5.4. E. H. Bradley, B. R. Elkins, J. Herrin, and B. Elbel, "Health and Social Services Expenditures: Associations with Health Outcomes," *BMJ Safety and Quality* 20, no. 10 (2011): 826–831, fig. 1. Adapted with permission of Elizabeth Bradley.

Figure 6.1. US Department of Health and Human Services, *The Health Consequences of Smoking—50 Years of Progress: A Report of the Surgeon General* (Atlanta, GA: US Dept. of Health and Human Services, Centers for Disease Control and Prevention, National Center for Chronic Disease Prevention and Health Promotion, Office on Smoking and Health, 2014), fig. 2.1.

Figure 7.1. Data source: D. M. Berwick and A. D. Hackbarth, "Eliminating Waste in US Health Care," *JAMA* 307 (April 11, 2012): 1513–1516.

Index